T0263210

Castleman Disease

Editors

FRITS VAN RHEE
NIKHIL C. MUNSHI

HEMATOLOGY/ONCOLOGY CLINICS OF NORTH AMERICA

www.hemonc.theclinics.com

Consulting Editors
GEORGE P. CANELLOS
H. FRANKLIN BUNN

February 2018 • Volume 32 • Number 1

ELSEVIER

1600 John F. Kennedy Boulevard • Suite 1800 • Philadelphia, Pennsylvania, 19103-2899

http://www.theclinics.com

HEMATOLOGY/ONCOLOGY CLINICS OF NORTH AMERICA Volume 32, Number 1
February 2018 ISSN 0889-8588, ISBN 13: 978-0-323-58289-6

Editor: Stacy Eastman
Developmental Editor: Kristen Helm

Photocopying
Single photocopies of single articles may be made for personal use as allowed by national copyright laws. Permission of the Publisher and payment of a fee is required for all other photocopying, including multiple or systematic copying, copying for advertising or promotional purposes, resale, and all forms of document delivery. Special rates are available for educational institutions that wish to make photocopies for non-profit educational classroom use. For information on how to seek permission visit www.elsevier.com/permissions or call: (+44) 1865 843830 (UK)/(+1) 215 239 3804 (USA).

Derivative Works
Subscribers may reproduce tables of contents or prepare lists of articles including abstracts for internal circulation within their institutions. Permission of the Publisher is required for resale or distribution outside the institution. Permission of the Publisher is required for all other derivative works, including compilations and translations (please consult www.elsevier.com/permissions).

Electronic Storage or Usage
Permission of the Publisher is required to store or use electronically any material contained in this periodical, including any article or part of an article (please consult www.elsevier.com/permissions). Except as outlined above, no part of this publication may be reproduced, stored in a retrieval system or transmitted in any form or by any means, electronic, mechanical, photocopying, recording or otherwise, without prior written permission of the Publisher.

Notice
No responsibility is assumed by the Publisher for any injury and/or damage to persons or property as a matter of products liability, negligence or otherwise, or from any use or operation of any methods, products, instructions or ideas contained in the material herein. Because of rapid advances in the medical sciences, in particular, independent verification of diagnoses and drug dosages should be made.

Although all advertising material is expected to conform to ethical (medical) standards, inclusion in this publication does not constitute a guarantee or endorsement of the quality or value of such product or of the claims made of it by its manufacturer.

Hematology/Oncology Clinics (ISSN 0889-8588) is published bimonthly by Elsevier Inc., 360 Park Avenue South, New York, NY 10010-1710. Months of issue are February, April, June, August, October, and December. Business and Editorial Offices: 1600 John F. Kennedy Blvd., Ste. 1800, Philadelphia, PA 19103—2899. Customer Service Office: 3251 Riverport Lane, Maryland Heights, MO 63043. Periodicals postage paid at New York, NY and at additional mailing offices. Subscription prices are $413.00 per year (domestic individuals), $787.00 per year (domestic institutions), $100.00 per year (domestic students/residents), $471.00 per year (Canadian individuals), $974.00 per year (Canadian institutions) $536.00 per year (international individuals), $974.00 per year (international institutions), and $255.00 per year (international and Canadian students/residents). International air speed delivery is included in all *Clinics* subscription prices. All prices are subject to change without notice. **POSTMASTER:** Send address changes to *Hematology/Oncology Clinics of North America*, Elsevier Health Sciences Division, Subscription Customer Service, 3251 Riverport Lane, Maryland Heights, MO 63043. Customer Service (orders, claims, online, change of address): Elsevier Health Sciences Division, Subscription **Customer Service, 3251 Riverport Lane, Maryland Heights, MO 63043. Tel: 1-800-654-2452 (U.S. and Canada); 314-447-8871 (outside U.S. and Canada). Fax: 314-447-8029. E-mail: journalscustomerservice-usa@elsevier.com (for print support); journalsonlinesupport-usa@elsevier.com (for online support).**

Reprints. For copies of 100 or more, of articles in this publication, please contact the Commercial Reprints Department, Elsevier Inc., 360 Park Avenue South, New York, New York 10010-1710; Tel.: 212-633-3874, Fax: 212-633-3820, E-mail: reprints@elsevier.com.

Hematology/Oncology Clinics of North America is covered in *MEDLINE/PubMed (Index Medicus)*, *EMBASE/ Excerpta Medica, and BIOSIS.*

Contributors

CONSULTING EDITORS

GEORGE P. CANELLOS, MD
William Rosenberg Professor of Medicine, Department of Medical Oncology, Dana-Farber Cancer Institute, Boston, Massachusetts, USA

H. FRANKLIN BUNN, MD
Professor of Medicine, Division of Hematology, Brigham and Women's Hospital, Harvard Medical School, Boston, Massachusetts, USA

EDITORS

FRITS VAN RHEE, MD, PhD, MRCP(UK), FRCPath, FACP
Professor of Medicine, Director of Developmental and Translational Medicine, Charles and Clydene Scharlau Chair of Hematological Malignancies Research, UAMS Myeloma Institute, University of Arkansas for Medical Sciences, Little Rock, Arkansas, USA

NIKHIL C. MUNSHI, MD
Professor of Medicine, Harvard Medical School, Director, Basic and Correlative Sciences, Associate Director, Jerome Lipper Myeloma Center, Medical Oncology, Dana-Farber Cancer Institute, Boston, Massachusetts, USA; VA Boston Healthcare System, West Roxbury, Massachusetts, USA

AUTHORS

FRANCIS BUADI, MD
Assistant Professor, Medicine, Mayo Clinic, Rochester, Minnesota, USA

ANGELA DISPENZIERI, MD
Professor, Medicine, Mayo Clinic, Rochester, Minnesota, USA

DAVID C. FAJGENBAUM, MD, MBA, MSc
Assistant Professor of Medicine, Associate Director, Patient Impact, Penn Orphan Disease Center, Division of Translational Medicine and Human Genetics, Hospital of the University of Pennsylvania, Philadelphia, Pennsylvania, USA

AMY GREENWAY, BS, CRS
Research Associate, UAMS Myeloma Institute, University of Arkansas for Medical Sciences, Little Rock, Arkansas, USA

TAKURO IGAWA, MD
Department of Pathology, Okayama University Graduate School of Medicine, Dentistry and Pharmaceutical Sciences, Okayama, Japan

HIROKI ITO
Department of Biomolecular Science and Regulation, The Institute of Scientific and Industrial Research, Osaka University, Ibaraki, Osaka, Japan

ARNAUD JACCARD, MD, PhD
Department of Clinical Hematology, Reference Center for AL Amyloidosis, CHU, Limoges, France

ELAINE S. JAFFE, MD
Laboratory of Pathology, Hematopathology Section, Center for Cancer Research, National Cancer Institute, Bethesda, Maryland, USA

TOMOHIRO KOGA, MD, PhD
Assistant Professor, Department of Immunology and Rheumatology, Division of Advanced Preventive Medical Sciences, Assistant Professor, Center for Bioinformatics and Molecular Medicine, Graduate School of Biomedical Sciences, Nagasaki University, Nagasaki, Japan

TAXIARCHIS KOURELIS, MD
Assistant Professor, Medicine, Mayo Clinic, Rochester, Minnesota, USA

MEGAN S. LIM, MD, PhD
Department of Pathology and Laboratory Medicine, Perelman School of Medicine University of Pennsylvania, Philadelphia, Pennsylvania, USA

KATHRYN LURAIN, MD, MPH
HIV and AIDS Malignancy Branch, Center for Cancer Research, National Cancer Institute, Bethesda, Maryland, USA

MICHELLE L. MAUERMANN, MD
Associate Professor, Department of Neurology, Mayo Clinic, Rochester, Minnesota, USA

NIKHIL C. MUNSHI, MD
Professor of Medicine, Harvard Medical School, Director, Basic and Correlative Sciences, Associate Director, Jerome Lipper Myeloma Center, Medical Oncology, Dana-Farber Cancer Institute, Boston, Massachusetts, USA; VA Boston Healthcare System, West Roxbury, Massachusetts, USA

SHINICHI MURAYAMA, PhD
Department of Biomolecular Science and Regulation, The Institute of Scientific and Industrial Research, Osaka University, Ibaraki, Osaka, Japan

YASUHARU SATO, MD
Department of Pathology, Okayama University Graduate School of Medicine, Dentistry and Pharmaceutical Sciences, Division of Pathophysiology, Graduate School of Health Sciences/Faculty of Health Sciences, Okayama University, Okayama, Japan

DUSTIN SHILLING, PhD
Associate Director, Castleman Research Program, Division of Translational Medicine and Human Genetics, Hospital of the University of Pennsylvania, Philadelphia, Pennsylvania, USA

DAVID SIMPSON, MBChB, FRACP, FRCPA
Haematologist, North Shore Hospital, Auckland, New Zealand

KATIE STONE, BS, CRS
Laboratory Director, UAMS Myeloma Institute, University of Arkansas for Medical Sciences, Little Rock, Arkansas, USA

RAPHAËL SZALAT, MD
Medical Oncology, Dana-Farber Cancer Institute, Harvard Medical School, Boston, Massachusetts, USA

THOMAS S. ULDRICK, MD, MS
HIV and AIDS Malignancy Branch, Center for Cancer Research, National Cancer Institute, Bethesda, Maryland, USA

FRITS VAN RHEE, MD, PhD, MRCP(UK), FRCPath, FACP
Professor of Medicine, Director of Developmental and Translational Medicine, Charles and Clydene Scharlau Chair of Hematological Malignancies Research, UAMS Myeloma Institute, University of Arkansas for Medical Sciences, Little Rock, Arkansas, USA

RAYMOND S.M. WONG, MBChB, MD
Clinical Associate Professor (Honorary), Department of Medicine and Therapeutics, Sir Y.K. Pao Cancer Centre, Prince of Wales Hospital, The Chinese University of Hong Kong, Shatin, New Territories, Hong Kong

DAVID WU, MD, PhD
Department of Laboratory Medicine, University of Washington, Seattle, Washington, USA

ROBERT YARCHOAN, MD
HIV and AIDS Malignancy Branch, Center for Cancer Research, National Cancer Institute, Bethesda, Maryland, USA

KAZUYUKI YOSHIZAKI, MD, PhD
Professor, Department of Biomolecular Science and Regulation, The Institute of Scientific and Industrial Research, Osaka University, Ibaraki, Osaka, Japan

Contents

Castleman disease is a rare entity, including unicentric Castleman disease (UCD), human herpesvirus-8 plus Castleman disease (HHV-8+MCD), and idiopathic multicentric Castleman disease (iMCD). UCD is the most common at 16 per million person-years and occurs at every age. HHV-8+MCD incidence varies widely, mostly affecting human immunodeficiency virus–positive men. iMCD is likely a more heterogeneous disease with an estimated incidence of 5 per million person-years. Improved definitions should improve understanding of the epidemiology of Castleman disease and its subtypes.

Castleman disease (CD) describes a group of heterogeneous disorders with common lymph node histopathologic features, including atrophic or hyperplastic germinal centers, prominent follicular dendritic cells, hypervascularization, polyclonal lymphoproliferation, and/or polytypic plasmacytosis. The cause and pathogenesis of the four subtypes of CD (unicentric CD; human herpesvirus-8-associated multicentric CD; polyradiculoneuropathy, organomegaly, endocrinopathy, monoclonal plasma cell disorder, and skin changes [POEMS]–associated multicentric CD; and idiopathic multicentric CD) vary considerably. This article provides a summary of our current understanding of the cause, cell types, signaling pathways, and effector cytokines implicated in the pathogenesis of each subtype.

Since the discovery of Castleman disease, improvements in treating the disease and its variants have centered on interleukin-6 (IL-6). IL-6 was discovered from T-cell factors (BCDF or BSF-2), which induced B-cell maturation. Most symptoms of the plasma cell variant of Castleman disease are linked to the hyperfunction of IL-6, constitutively produced in the affected lymph nodes (1989), suggesting IL-6 is key in the pathogenesis of multicentric Castleman disease (MCD). The results of several studies have shown that most MCD symptoms and abnormal laboratory results are improved by anti-IL-6 MCD treatments, such as tocilizumab, a humanized anti-IL-6 receptor antibody, and siltuximab, an anti-IL-6 antibody.

The term Castleman disease encompasses several distinct lymphoproliferative disorders with different underlying disease pathogenesis and clinical outcomes. It includes unicentric and multicentric diseases with limited versus significant systemic symptoms, respectively. Importantly, the histopathologic features encountered in the various forms of Castleman disease are diverse and, for the most part, lack specificity, because they are seen to varying degrees in different clinical variants of Castleman disease and in reactive (autoimmune or infectious) and malignant (lymphoma) contexts. Accordingly, accurate clinical diagnosis of Castleman disease requires careful and thorough clinicopathologic correlation. An overview of the key histopathologic features of Castleman disease is presented.

Castleman disease (CD) is a rare and heterogenous group of disorders sharing in common an abnormal lymph node pathology. CD comprises distinct subtypes with different prognoses. Unicentric CD and multicentric CD are featured by specific systemic manifestations and may be associated with Kaposi sarcoma, non-Hodgkin and Hodgkin lymphoma, and POEMS syndrome. Multicentric CD is classically associated with systemic symptoms and poorer prognosis. In this article, the authors review how to diagnose the disease, keeping in context the clinical findings, biochemical changes, and complications associated with CD.

Unicentric Castleman disease (UCD) is a rare lymphoproliferative disorder that manifests typically as proliferation of a single lymph node or region of lymph nodes. Histologically, hyaline vascular variant is found in a majority of UCDs. UCD commonly presents in younger patient populations. Patients with UCD may be asymptomatic or present with symptoms related to mass effects on surrounding structures. It is difficult to achieve a definitive diagnosis by imaging alone. Histologic examination of the lesion remains the gold standard for diagnosis. Complete surgical resection is the best primary treatment modality for UCD resulting in excellent long-term survival and low recurrence rates.

Kaposi sarcoma herpesvirus (KSHV)-associated multicentric Castleman disease (MCD) is a rare, polyclonal lymphoproliferative disorder characterized by flares of inflammatory symptoms, edema, cytopenias, lymphadenopathy, and splenomegaly. Diagnosis requires a lymph node biopsy. Pathogenesis is related to dysregulated inflammatory cytokines, including human and viral interleukin-6. Rituximab alone or in combination with chemotherapy, such as liposomal doxorubicin, has led to an overall survival of over 90% at 5 years. Experimental approaches to treatment include virus-activated cytotoxic therapy with high-dose zidovudine and valganciclovir and targeting human interleukin-6 activity. Despite successful treatment of KSHV-MCD, patients remain at high risk for developing non-Hodgkin lymphomas.

directed at the underlying plasma cell clone with risk-adapted therapy based on the extent of the plasma cell disorder. Radiation therapy is effective for patients with a localized presentation, without bone marrow involvement, and 1 to 3 bone lesions. Patients with disseminated disease should receive, preferably, high-dose chemotherapy with peripheral blood transplantation. Low-dose melphalan and dexamethasone or new agents used in myeloma are also effective. The most promising agent is lenalidomide, which could be given before high-dose therapy or radiation to get rapid neurologic responses.

Polyneuropathy, organomegaly, endocrinopathy, monoclonal plasma cell disorder, and skin changes (POEMS) syndrome is a rare paraneoplastic disorder. The polyneuropathy can be the presenting symptom and is typically a painful, motor-predominant polyradiculoneuropathy often mimicking chronic inflammatory demyelinating polyradiculoneuropathy. The presence of a lambda monoclonal protein, elevated vascular endothelial growth factor, systemic features, and treatment resistance are clues to the diagnosis. Castleman disease (CD) is seen in a subset of these patients, and when present the neuropathy is similar but less severe. In contrast, in those patients with purely CD, the neuropathy is often a mild, painless distal sensory neuropathy.

HEMATOLOGY/ONCOLOGY CLINICS OF NORTH AMERICA

ISSUE OF RELATED INTEREST

Medical Clinics of North America, March 2017 (Vol. 101, Issue 2)
Anemia
Thomas G. DeLoughery, *Editor*
Available at: http://www.medical.theclinics.com/

THE CLINICS ARE AVAILABLE ONLINE!
Access your subscription at:
www.theclinics.com

Preface

Castleman Disease

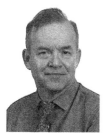 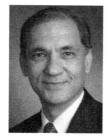

Frits van Rhee, MD, PhD, MRCP(UK),   Nikhil C. Munshi, MD
FRCPath, FACP

Editors

In the course of studying tumors of the thymus gland we came across a small group of cases in which enlarged mediastinal lymph nodes resembled thymic tumors grossly, radiologically and even microscopically …[1]

In 1954, Dr Benjamin Castleman first described a rare and enigmatic disease that now carries his name. Over the past 60 years, this disease has captivated researchers, who have come to recognize unicentric and multicentric varieties and have uncovered different pathologic entities of the condition. Though these discoveries have led to more questions, it is clear that for some patients the disease is driven by the HHV8 (human herpes virus 8) virus, which produces a separate clinicopathologic entity requiring a specific type of therapy, while others suffer from an idiopathic form of multicentric Castleman disease (iMCD). Although the cause of this form of the disease remains unknown, it is evident that interleukin-6 (IL-6) plays a critical role in the pathophysiology. This discovery led to the development of novel anti-IL-6 monoclonal antibodies and the first approved therapies for iMCD. However, not all patients benefit from these innovations, and other distinct entities have recently been described, such as TAFRO (thrombocytopenia, anasarca, fever, renal dysfunction, reticulin fibrosis, and organomegaly) syndrome, which may prove to have its own unique cytokine profile. Others have disease that occurs in coexistence or partial overlap with POEMS syndrome.

Through a collaborative effort, researchers and clinicians from all over the world have joined in the Castleman Disease Collaborative Network to create, prioritize, and implement a research agenda based on new hypotheses, gather real-life data pertaining to epidemiology, clinical features, and treatment response as well as establish a biobank for research. In addition, the first consensus diagnostic criteria were published in 2016.

Hematol Oncol Clin N Am 32 (2018) xiii–xiv
https://doi.org/10.1016/j.hoc.2017.10.001
0889-8588/18/© 2017 Published by Elsevier Inc.

hemonc.theclinics.com

In this issue, experts in the field have provided latest information pertaining to all aspects of the disease, including epidemiology, pathogenetic mechanisms, histopathology, and diagnosis of iMCD. In addition to which, there is focus on treatments for patients with unicentric Castleman disease, iMCD, HHV8-associated multicentric Castleman disease, and the recently described TAFRO syndrome. A special emphasis is given to information regarding POEMS syndrome, a condition related to Castleman disease.

We thank the authors from all over the world for their valuable contributions. We are proud to present the first issue ever dedicated to Castleman disease and hope that it will be a unique and valuable source of information for both Castleman disease and POEMS syndrome.

Frits van Rhee, MD, PhD, MRCP(UK), FRCPath, FACP
Myeloma Institute
University of Arkansas for Medical Sciences
4301 West Markham, #816
Little Rock, AR 72205, USA

Nikhil C. Munshi, MD
Dana Farber Cancer Institute
VA Boston Healthcare System
Harvard Medical School
450 Brookline Avenue, M230
Boston, MA 02215, USA

E-mail addresses:
vanrheefrits@uams.edu (F. van Rhee)
nikhil_munshi@dfci.harvard.edu (N.C. Munshi)

REFERENCE

1. Castleman B, Iverson L, Menendez VP. Localized mediastinal lymphnode hyperplasia resembling thymoma. Cancer 1956;9(4):822–30.

Epidemiology of Castleman Disease

David Simpson, MBChB, FRACP, FRCPA

KEYWORDS

- Unicentric Castleman • Multicentric Castleman • TAFRO • HHV-8

KEY POINTS

- The incidence of unicentric Castleman disease is 15 per million patient years.
- The incidence of idiopathic multicentric Castleman disease is 5 per million patient years, but with regional variation.
- Human herpesvirus-8 (HHV-8) plus multicentric Castleman disease is most common in men infected with HHV-8 HIV and is more common in the era of highly active antiretroviral therapy.

Accurate assessment of the epidemiology of Castleman disease (CD) has been hampered by lack of an International Statistical Classification of Diseases and Related Health Problems (ICD) code and no formal definition of the disease. However, the ICD code (ICD-10-CM D47.Z2), which became effective on October 1, 2016, and published the diagnostic criteria,[1] will allow improved data regarding this of the cluster of diseases that make up this rare entity. Estimates of the incidence of CD vary widely. In an attempt to better determine the incidence, a systematic search of a claims database was undertaken.[2] Two commercial insurance claims databases, IMS LifeLink and Truven Health Analytics MarketScan, which together include medical records on nearly 200 million people, were screened for patients with an index diagnosis of lymphadenopathy (ICD-9 code 785.6) who were enrolled for 1 year before or 2 years after the index diagnosis. This was done to ensure that there was an opportunity to meet the CD characteristics as published in 2005.[3] Patients were excluded if they did not have a lymph node biopsy because this is required for CD diagnosis. Those with rheumatoid arthritis, lupus, cancer (including lymphoma), and human immunodeficiency virus (HIV) were also excluded. The estimated incidence rate for CD was 21 (IMS LifeLink) to 25 (MarketScan) per million person-years. Applying this rate to the US population 25 years and older (assumed to be 207,301,600 in 2011), the incidence of CD in the United States is 4353 to 5183 patients. To try to estimate the proportion of these patients who had multicentric CD (MCD), MCD was assumed to be the

Disclosures: I have previously received an honorarium from Janssen.
North Shore Hospital, Private Bag 93-503, Takapuna, Auckland 0740, New Zealand
E-mail address: david.simpson@waitematadhb.govt.nz

Hematol Oncol Clin N Am 32 (2018) 1–10
https://doi.org/10.1016/j.hoc.2017.09.001
0889-8588/18/© 2017 Elsevier Inc. All rights reserved.

diagnosis if patients had been treated with doxorubicin, dexamethasone, prednisone, or rituximab, which are drugs that were commonly given for MCD between 2001 and 2009, the years analyzed in the review.[4] It was estimated that 23% of patients with CD were potentially suffering from MCD, equating to 1001 to 1192 cases in the United States, with the other 77% assumed to have unicentric CD (UCD). There are several assumptions in this algorithm, hence the confidence limits of this estimate remain very wide. However, the numbers estimated are remarkably similar to those obtained using other methodologies.

An alternative approach to estimate the incidence of MCD in the Asia-Pacific region involved a survey of centers in Southeast Victoria (Monash Health System), Australia (subsample number [n] = 10); Hong Kong, China (n = 1); and Auckland, New Zealand (n = 1). This produced an average MCD point prevalence estimate of about 5 per million.[5] All regions surveyed had similar estimates ranging from 4.2 to 5.4 per million. The proportion of cases that are multicentric can vary by ethnicity and higher rates are reported in Polynesians living in New Zealand[6] (see later discussion).

The 3 main broad subtypes of CD each have distinctive etiologic factors and so it is important to consider them separately. These include (1) UCD, (2) human herpesvirus-8 (HHV-8) plus MCD (HHV-8+MCD), and (3) idiopathic MCD (iMCD). In addition to these broad groups, there seem to be other distinct subtypes of iMCD. These include (1) polyradiculoneuropathy, organomegaly, endocrinopathy, monoclonal plasma cell neoplasm, and skin changes (POEMS) related MCD; and (2) thrombocytopenia, anasarca, fever, renal insufficiency, and organomegaly (TAFRO) syndrome. The term oligocentric or regional CD has also been proposed for a subtype of UCD with clusters of regionally confined nodes.[7]

UNICENTRIC CASTLEMAN DISEASE

UCD can present at any age, from the very young to the elderly, but it predominantly presents at a younger age than MCD. A literature review was performed to identify reported cases of CD and was published in 2012.[8] Of 404 cases, 274 or 68% had UCD. The median age at presentation was 34 years with a wide age range (2–84 years) and a mild female predominance (60%). This is almost identical to a North American series of 54 patients from the Mayo clinic and the University of Nebraska (**Fig. 1**). The median age in this series was 34 years (range 4–74 years), including 4 cases in patients younger than 10 years of age.[9] Additional cases have been reported in children as young as 2 years of age.[10] A series from Beijing, China, of 145 HIV-negative patients, clinically classified 69 (47.6%) cases as UCD[11] (**Fig. 2**). The median age was 40 years for the whole group, with an even sex distribution (52% female).

UCD is thought to be rare, with no reliable estimates of its incidence in the population (to date). The insurance claims database screening study estimated the rate at 16 per million.[2] Smaller case series have the potential for referral bias because MCD cases are more difficult to manage and more likely to be referred to a center of excellence, skewing the relative proportion of the 2 entities. There seems to be similar incidence and pattern of disease in series reported from the United States,[9] China,[11] Czechoslovakia,[12] Japan,[13] and New Zealand.[6]

A small number of cases, perhaps 5% to 10% of UCD, present with regionally clustered nodes. These patients more often have systemic symptoms of anemia, high C-reactive protein (CRP), and low albumin, in keeping with high levels of interleukin (IL)-6. Immunoglobulins are not increased. Seen in both younger and older patients, there are insufficient data to determine if this is a different entity and the incidence, sex, and age distribution.

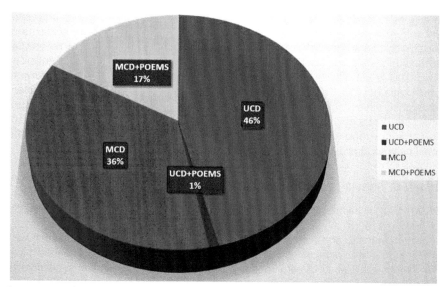

Fig. 1. Mayo Clinic and the University of Nebraska CD cases. *Data from* Dispenzieri A, Armitage JO, Loe MJ, et al. The clinical spectrum of Castleman's disease. Am J Hematol 2012;87(11):997-1002.

About 95% of cases of UCD cases have hyaline vascular histology.[9,14] There is not enough evidence to determine if other histologic subtypes, mixed histology, or plasma cell variants, have different epidemiology. The cause of UCD remains unknown but there is accumulating evidence it is a clonal disorder. Chang and

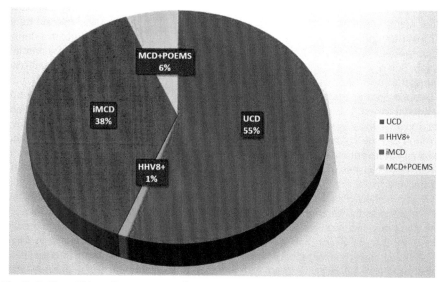

Fig. 2. Beijing, China, CD cases. *Data from* Zhang L, Li Z, Cao X, et al. Clinical spectrum and survival analysis of 145 cases of HIV-negative Castleman's disease: renal function is an important prognostic factor. Sci Rep 2016;6:23831.

colleagues[15] used the human androgen receptor-α (HUMARA) gene to assess clonality in female patients with unicentric hyaline vascular CD. They found evidence of clonality but no evidence of immunoglobulin and T-cell receptor gene rearrangements, suggesting the clonal cell is likely to be of stromal or follicular dendritic cell origin. This is supported by the development of follicular dendritic cell sarcoma in some cases of UCD. This is a rare entity that makes up 0.4% of sarcomas. A recent series of 66 cases, showed 6 subjects also had hyaline vascular variant CD: 2 subjects were diagnosed with CD before their sarcoma and 4 subjects had both diagnoses made concurrently.[16] It is possible the sarcomas represent transformation of a clonal cell responsible for the development of UCD.

HUMAN HERPESVIRUS-8 PLUS MULTICENTRIC CASTLEMAN DISEASE

HHV-8+MCD is the most clearly defined and understood variant of CD. HHV-8+MCD is a waxing and waning acute febrile illness characterized by diffuse lymphadenopathy, splenomegaly, and anemia. By definition, HHV-8+MVD requires infection with HHV-8. HHV-8 was originally discovered in 1994, when Chang and colleagues[17] isolated herpesvirus-like DNA sequences from Kaposi sarcoma lesions in subjects with AIDS. By comparing tumor and constitutional DNA, they found the additional DNA sequences that corresponded to a new herpesvirus. This was initially called Kaposi sarcoma–associated herpesvirus (KSHV) but later classified as HHV-8. HHV-8 is a rhadinovirus, a genus that have mastered the ability to pirate cellular genes from their host cells and incorporate them into their genomes.[18] For example, most rhadinoviruses have a copy of the cyclin gene, which regulates the ability of the cell to divide. In the case of HHV-8, 1 co-opted gene is the viral homologue of IL-6 (vIL-6). Most of this genus infect animals and generally cause tumors only when infection occurs outside of their native hosts. HHV-8, however, resides in humans and causes cancers when the host is immunosuppressed, most often due to HIV coinfection, old age, or following organ transplantation.

The seroprevalence of HHV-8 has significant global heterogeneity. In contrast to other members of the herpesvirus family that infect most humans, the infection rates in most parts of the world are low. In northern Europe, Southeast Asia, and the Caribbean the seroprevalence is around 2% to 4%.[19] In Mediterranean populations (ie, Israel, Saudi Arabia, Italy, and Greece), rates are higher at approximately 10%; whereas, in sub-Saharan Africa, prevalence rates are highest at around 40%.[20]

Despite greater understanding of this virus, the methods of transmission are not well-established. It is spread sexually; however, the sexual acts of greatest risk are not known. The observation of high seroprevalence in prepubertal children residing in Africa and the Western and Eastern Mediterranean regions suggests other epidemiologically relevant routes of transmission.[21,22] Data from HHV-8 mothers in Gabon found very low rates of HHV-8 DNA in cord blood, suggesting transmission occurs after delivery.[23]

HHV-8 is shed in saliva. HHV-8 DNA was detected in saliva from 14 out of 35 (40%) HIV-infected individuals and 4 out of 35 (11.4%) non-HIV-infected individuals.[24,25] Shedding in saliva requires the virus to be in the lytic phase, and the virus is mostly found in the saliva of immunocompromised individuals.[26] Conversely, in HIV-coinfected hosts, the cluster of differentiation 4 (CD4) count is the most important predictor of HHV-8 salivary shedding, with increased prevalence of HHV-8 salivary DNA at higher CD4 counts. The odds of salivary HHV-8 shedding at CD4 counts greater than or equal to 350 cells/μL was 63 times the odds of shedding at CD4 less than 350.[24] HHV-8 is also present in the mononuclear cells in semen and in sperm from

HIV-coinfected individuals[27]; however, it is absent from semen in immunocompetent hosts. The importance of semen in spreading the virus is unclear.

Given the coexistence of HHV-8 and HIV,[28] the largest immunocompromised population with HHV-8+MCD is HIV-positive. A systematic literature review of subjects diagnosed with HIV and HHV-8+MCD[29] found that, out of 84 cases, 48 were on highly active antiretroviral therapy (HAART), and 31 of these subjects were on HAART at the time of MCD diagnosis. These subjects had a better immunologic profile and a lower incidence of Kaposi sarcoma than those who initiated HAART after MCD diagnosis. Surprisingly, unlike Kaposi sarcoma whose incidence has reduced in the HAART era, HHV-8+MCD has increased. Looking at a large prospective database of HIV-positive individuals, 24 with HHV-8+MCD were identified. The incidence in the pre-HAART (1983–1996), early-HAART (1997–2001), and later HAART (2002–2007) eras were 2.3 (95% CI 0.02–4.2), 2.8 (95% CI 0.9–6.5) and 8.3 (95% CI 4.6–12.6), respectively, representing a statistically significant increase over time ($P < .05$).[30] Multivariate analysis demonstrated that a nadir CD4 count greater than 200/mm, increased age, no previous HAART exposure, and non-white ethnicity were all associated with an increased risk of MCD.

IDIOPATHIC MULTICENTRIC CASTLEMAN DISEASE

iMCD is an entity of unknown cause. Possible causes include a virus other than HHV-8, paracrine secretion of cytokines by a small population of neoplastic cells, autoinflammatory mechanisms, or genetic defects in IL-6 regulation.[31] It is possible, or rather probable, that there is more than 1 cause because this subgroup of CD is more heterogeneous than the others. POEMS-associated iMCD and TAFRO are considered separately (see later discussion). The claims database review suggested the incidence of HIV-negative MCD was 5 per million,[2] supported by an Asian-Pacific survey.[5] The relative proportion of cases of MCD that belong in the idiopathic category varies between case series, probably reflecting referral biases of the specialist groups.

Series reported from HIV treatment centers have a much larger proportion of cases that have HHV-8+MCD.[32,33] A series of 16 cases from single center in India showed 8 cases each of were UCD and MVD, no cases were HIV-positive.

The median age of presentation is older in iMCD cases compared with UCD. The Mayo Clinic and University of Nebraska reported data on 60 patients with MCD and showed that 32% had criteria sufficient for a diagnosis of POEMS syndrome.[9] This is higher than other reports and likely reflects referral bias. In the non-POEMS iMCD patients the median age was 51 years (range 16–78 years), with an equal sex ratio (female 51%). A review of published surgical cases identified 126 patients with MCD, the median age was similar at 50 years (range 1–83 years) and higher than the UCD cohort median 33.8 years (range 2–84 years). In contrast there was a strong male predominance (female 38%) compared with UCD (female 59%). HIV patients were not included, but there were 46 out of 126 cases with MCD who were HHV-8 positive, which is in contrast to other series; for example, only 1 out of 76 cases in the Beijing series were HHV-8 positive. The demographics of the HHV-8 patients were analyzed separately.

POLYNESIAN IDIOPATHIC MULTICENTRIC CASTLEMAN DISEASE

There is an increased prevalence of CD in Polynesians living in New Zealand.[6] At the author's center within Auckland, New Zealand, the Waitemata District Health Board, we service a population of 600,000 (597,510 population estimate 2016–2017). In unpublished data from the patient database, we have 17 cases of CD equating to a prevalence of 28 per million, including 6 with UCD (including 2 with oligocentric presentation), and 11 with iMCD (including 1 POEMS). The MCD to UCD ratio (65%) is higher than reported elsewhere, with a notable Polynesian predominance among iMCD patients with 8 Polynesians (73%; New Zealand Maori 4, Samoan 3, Niuean 1) and 3 Europeans. Polynesians make up 17% of the population or about 102,000, making the incidence of iMCD in Polynesians 80 per million. To determine if there were other undiagnosed cases, we performed a search of the hospital laboratory records for patients who had an IgG level greater than 35 g/L over a 3-year period. We identified a further 3 cases of possible CD, all in Polynesians; however, no patients were available for confirmation of diagnosis.[6] There are fewer data from the rest of New Zealand, but it is appreciated that most patients seen with iMCD are Polynesians. There have been no cases reported in relatives of those with iMCD, but the striking rate seen in Polynesians suggest a genetic predisposition to this disease. Their presentation is characterized by anemia, high CRP, marked polyclonal increase in immunoglobulins, and cutaneous lesions that can be very extensive, similar to a series reported from Japan.[34] The prognosis is favorable with all treated patients responding to IL-6 blockade, using tocilizumab or siltuximab. There are genetic similarities between Taiwanese, Filipinos, and Polynesians.[35] Recent DNA evidence has confirmed that the early Polynesians who populated the islands of the South Pacific migrated around 3000 BP and originated from indigenous Amis Taiwanese (**Fig. 3**).

POLYRADICULONEUROPATHY, ORGANOMEGALY, ENDOCRINOPATHY, MONOCLONAL PLASMA CELL NEOPLASM, AND SKIN CHANGES RELATED TO IDIOPATHIC MULTICENTRIC CASTLEMAN DISEASE

POEMS syndrome is a paraneoplastic syndrome.[36] The important features, other than those in its previously listed acronym, include papilledema, extravascular volume overload, sclerotic bone lesions, thrombocytosis, elevated vascular endothelial growth factor (VEGF), and abnormal pulmonary function.[37] By definition, it is

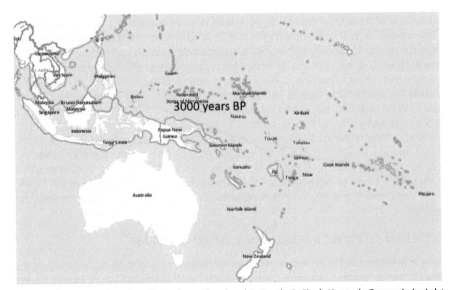

Fig. 3. Polynesian migration. *Data from* Skoglund P, Posth C, Sirak K, et al. Genomic insights into the peopling of the Southwest Pacific. Nature 2016;538(7626):510-3.

associated with monoclonal plasma cell disorder that, in most cases, is lambda light chain restricted. The relevance of the lambda light chain restriction is unclear but it is interesting that HHV-8 only infects lambda plasmablasts,[38] although this may be coincidental. The treatment of POEMS is mainly to target the plasma cell clone using myeloma therapy.[37] The incidence of POEMS is not well-defined but is about 5 per million. About 30% have CD as a clinical manifestation of their syndrome.[39] The proportion of MCD cases who have POEMS varies between case series. The Mayo Clinic and University of Nebraska reported data on 60 patients with MCD and showed 32% had criteria sufficient for a diagnosis of POEMS syndrome.[9] This is higher than other reports and likely reflects referral bias. The series from a single center in Beijing of 145 subjects with CD, found 69 subjects (47.6%) had UCD and 76 subjects (52.4%) had MCD, including 19 subjects (13.1%) who had POEMS.[11] Another series from a single center in Beijing of 114 subjects with CD found 52 (45.6%) with MCD and 7% who had POEMS.[14]

THROMBOCYTOPENIA, ANASARCA, FEVER, RENAL INSUFFICIENCY, AND ORGANOMEGALY

TAFRO syndrome is an acute or subacute systemic inflammatory disorder characterized by the conditions previously listed in the acronym. Of note, the anasarca includes pleural effusion and ascites and the organomegaly includes hepatosplenomegaly and lymphadenopathy.[40] It is a severe illness and often results in intensive care admission. Its cause is undetermined but it is associated with a cytokine storm with high levels of IL-6, VEGF, and other cytokines.[4,7] It was first described in a series of subjects from Japan in 2010.[41] Since then, similar cases have been recognized in other parts of the world.[31] Currently, most cases fit in the broader category of iMCD, although diagnostic criteria describing this as a separate entity have been published[40] and there seems to be distinct differences in its clinical features compared with classic CD.[31] There are very limited data on its incidence. In the Beijing series with 144 cases of CD, including 79 with MCD, only 1 subject (1.3%) fulfilled the diagnostic criteria of TAFRO.[11] In contrast, a series from MD Anderson found TAFRO subjects accounted for (9/43, 21%) subjects with iMCD, although this may represent referral bias.[42] The incidence of this is possibly about 2% of iMCD cases but this may vary geographically. Given that this disorder has only recently been defined, it is likely to some time before a truer appreciation of its incidence is gained.

SUMMARY

CD is a rare entity and, until recently, lacked an ICD code and diagnostic criteria. This has meant the true incidence estimates have varied widely. If clinicians are not familiar with this entity, patients may be labeled with other diagnoses; the degree to which this occurs is unknown. For UCD, there is nothing in the literature to suggest regional variation in the incidence and it can be seen in all age groups, including the very young. There is, perhaps, a subset of patients with regional adenopathy who are more likely to have raised inflammatory makers; these probably make up 5% to 10% of cases of UCD. Cases have been reported from several countries but there is little published information. The incidence of HHV-8+MCD varies widely because most patients with this form are HIV-positive men and cases are concentrated in HIV-treating centers. There are no data on rates in Africa where HHV-8 and HIV are prevalent. Prevalence rates do not seem to correlate with CD4 levels, and have not reduced with HAART, so it remains an important entity in HIV-positive populations. HHV-8+MCD can also be seen in non-HIV individuals. Although there are no data on the incidence of this, it is likely to show regional variation because HHV-8 prevalence is known to vary regionally. iMCD is likely a more heterogeneous disease. There seems to be racial differences in incidence, with high rates in Japan and in those with Polynesian ancestry. It is unclear if TAFRO represents a continuum of disease or is a distinct subtype of iMCD. The geographic location and racial make-up of a population likely determine the overall incidence and frequency of the different subentities. Although there has been much recent progress, with greater understanding and recognition of the disease, more light will be shed on the true epidemiology of CD and its subtypes.

REFERENCES

1. Fajgenbaum DC, Uldrick TS, Bagg A, et al. International, evidence-based consensus diagnostic criteria for HHV-8–negative/idiopathic multicentric Castleman disease. Blood 2017;129(12):1646.
2. Munshi N, Mehra M, van de Velde H, et al. Use of a claims database to characterize and estimate the incidence rate for Castleman disease. Leuk Lymphoma 2015;56(5):1252–60.
3. Casper C. The aetiology and management of Castleman disease at 50 years: translating pathophysiology to patient care. Br J Haematol 2005;129(1):3–17.
4. Liu AY, Nabel CS, Finkelman BS, et al. Idiopathic multicentric Castleman's disease: a systematic literature review. Lancet Haematol 2016;3(4):e163–75.
5. Katherine Heyland DRJ, Daniel T, Grima TS, et al. Preliminary prevalence estimate of multicentric Castleman's disease in Asia-Pacific. ISH; 2014.
6. Zhai S. Polynesian variant of idiopathic multicentric Castleman disease. Blood 2013;122(21):5127.
7. Fajgenbaum DC, van Rhee F, Nabel CS. HHV-8-negative, idiopathic multicentric Castleman disease: novel insights into biology, pathogenesis, and therapy. Blood 2014;123(19):2924.
8. Talat N, Belgaumkar AP, Schulte KM. Surgery in Castleman's disease: a systematic review of 404 published cases. Ann Surg 2012;255(4):677–84.
9. Dispenzieri A, Armitage JO, Loe MJ, et al. The clinical spectrum of Castleman's disease. Am J Hematol 2012;87(11):997–1002.
10. Linkhorn H, van der Meer G, Gruber M, et al. Castleman's disease: An unusually young presentation resulting in delayed diagnosis of a neck mass. Int J Pediatr Otorhinolaryngol 2016;86:90–2.
11. Zhang L, Li Z, Cao X, et al. Clinical spectrum and survival analysis of 145 cases of HIV-negative Castleman's disease: renal function is an important prognostic factor. Sci Rep 2016;6:23831.
12. Adam Z, Szturz P, Krejci M, et al. Treatment of 14 cases of Castlemans disease: the experience of one centre and an overview of literature. Vnitr Lek 2016;62(4):287–98 [in Czech].
13. Haro A, Kuramitsu E, Fukuyama Y. Complete resection of unicentric Castleman disease in the superior mediastinum: a case report. Int J Surg Case Rep 2016;25:44–7.
14. Dong Y, Wang M, Nong L, et al. Clinical and laboratory characterization of 114 cases of Castleman disease patients from a single centre: paraneoplastic pemphigus is an unfavourable prognostic factor. Br J Haematol 2015;169(6):834–42.
15. Chang KC, Wang YC, Hung LY, et al. Monoclonality and cytogenetic abnormalities in hyaline vascular Castleman disease. Mod Pathol 2014;27(6):823–31.

16. Jain P, Milgrom SA, Patel KP, et al. Characteristics, management, and outcomes of patients with follicular dendritic cell sarcoma. Br J Haematol 2017;178(3): 403–12.
17. Chang Y, Cesarman E, Pessin MS, et al. Identification of herpesvirus-like DNA sequences in AIDS-associated Kaposi's sarcoma. Science 1994;266(5192):1865–9.
18. Neipel F, Albrecht JC, Fleckenstein B. Cell-homologous genes in the Kaposi's sarcoma-associated rhadinovirus human herpesvirus 8: determinants of its pathogenicity? J Virol 1997;71(6):4187–92.
19. Zhang T, Wang L. Epidemiology of Kaposi's sarcoma-associated herpesvirus in Asia: Challenges and opportunities. J Med Virol 2017;89(4):563–70.
20. Chatlynne LG, Ablashi DV. Seroepidemiology of Kaposi's sarcoma-associated herpesvirus (KSHV). Semin Cancer Biol 1999;9(3):175–85.
21. Gessain A, Mauclere P, van Beveren M, et al. Human herpesvirus 8 primary infection occurs during childhood in Cameroon, Central Africa. Int J Cancer 1999; 81(2):189–92.
22. Pica F, Volpi A. Transmission of human herpesvirus 8: an update. Curr Opin Infect Dis 2007;20(2):152–6.
23. Capan-Melser M, Mombo-Ngoma G, Akerey-Diop D, et al. Epidemiology of human herpes virus 8 in pregnant women and their newborns–A cross-sectional delivery survey in Central Gabon. Int J Infect Dis 2015;39:16–9.
24. Gandhi M, Koelle DM, Ameli N, et al. Prevalence of human herpesvirus-8 salivary shedding in HIV increases with CD4 count. J Dental Res 2004;83(8):639–43.
25. de Franca TR, de Araujo RA, Ribeiro CM, et al. Salivary shedding of HHV-8 in people infected or not by human immunodeficiency virus 1. J Oral Pathol Med 2011;40(1):97–102.
26. Lucht E, Brytting M, Bjerregaard L, et al. Shedding of cytomegalovirus and herpesviruses 6, 7, and 8 in saliva of human immunodeficiency virus type 1-infected patients and healthy controls. Clin Infect Dis 1998;27(1):137–41.
27. Bagasra O, Patel D, Bobroski L, et al. Localization of human herpesvirus type 8 in human sperms by in situ PCR. J Mol Histol 2005;36(6–7):401–12.
28. Rohner E, Wyss N, Heg Z, et al. HIV and human herpesvirus 8 co-infection across the globe: Systematic review and meta-analysis. Int J Cancer 2016;138(1):45–54.
29. Mylona EE, Baraboutis IG, Lekakis LJ, et al. Multicentric Castleman's disease in HIV infection: a systematic review of the literature. AIDS Rev 2008;10(1):25–35.
30. Powles T, Stebbing J, Bazeos A, et al. The role of immune suppression and HHV-8 in the increasing incidence of HIV-associated multicentric Castleman's disease. Ann Oncol 2009;20(4):775–9.
31. Iwaki N, Fajgenbaum DC, Nabel CS, et al. Clinicopathologic analysis of TAFRO syndrome demonstrates a distinct subtype of HHV-8-negative multicentric Castleman disease. Am J Hematol 2016;91(2):220–6.
32. Uldrick TS, Polizzotto MN, Aleman K, et al. Rituximab plus liposomal doxorubicin in HIV-infected patients with KSHV-associated multicentric Castleman disease. Blood 2014;124(24):3544.
33. Oksenhendler E, Boulanger E, Galicier L, et al. High incidence of Kaposi sarcoma–associated herpesvirus–related non-Hodgkin lymphoma in patients with HIV infection and multicentric Castleman disease. Blood 2002;99(7):2331.
34. Kurosawa S, Akiyama N, Ohwada A, et al. Idiopathic plasmacytic lymphadenopathy with polyclonal hypergammaglobulinemia accompanied with cutaneous involvement and renal dysfunction. Jpn J Clin Oncol 2009;39(10):682–5.
35. Skoglund P, Posth C, Sirak K, et al. Genomic insights into the peopling of the Southwest Pacific. Nature 2016;538(7626):510–3.

36. Bardwick PA, Zvaifler NJ, Gill GN, et al. Plasma cell dyscrasia with polyneurop-athy, organomegaly, endocrinopathy, M protein, and skin changes: the POEMS syndrome. Report on two cases and a review of the literature. Medicine 1980; 59(4):311–22.
37. Dispenzieri A. How I treat POEMS syndrome. Blood 2012;119(24):5650–8.
38. Du MQ, Liu H, Diss TC, et al. Kaposi sarcoma-associated herpesvirus infects monotypic (IgM lambda) but polyclonal naive B cells in Castleman disease and associated lymphoproliferative disorders. Blood 2001;97(7):2130–6.
39. Dispenzieri A. POEMS syndrome: 2011 update on diagnosis, risk-stratification, and management. Am J Hematol 2011;86(7):591–601.
40. Masaki Y, Kawabata H, Takai K, et al. Proposed diagnostic criteria, disease severity classification and treatment strategy for TAFRO syndrome, 2015 version. Int J Hematol 2016;103(6):686–92.
41. Takai K, Nikkuni K, Shibuya H, et al. Thrombocytopenia with mild bone marrow fibrosis accompanied by fever, pleural effusion, ascites and hepatosplenome-galy. Rinsho ketsueki 2010;51(5):320–5 [in Japanese].
42. Yu L, Tu M, Cortes J, et al. Clinical and pathological characteristics of HIV- and HHV-8-negative Castleman disease. Blood 2017;129(12):1658–68.

Castleman Disease Pathogenesis

David C. Fajgenbaum, MD, MBA, MSc*, Dustin Shilling, PhD

KEYWORDS

- Castleman disease • Lymphoproliferative disorder • HHV-8 • POEMS • TAFRO
- Cytokine storm

KEY POINTS

- Castleman disease (CD) is subclassified based on the number of enlarged lymph nodes, Kaposi sarcoma–associated herpesvirus/human herpesvirus-8 (HHV-8) infection status, and clinical presentation.
- The pathogenesis of unicentric CD (adenopathy of a single region of lymph nodes) is most likely driven by a neoplastic follicular dendritic cell population.
- HHV-8–associated multicentric CD (adenopathy of multiple regions of lymph nodes) pathogenesis is virally driven, whereas polyneuropathy, organomegaly, endocrinopathy, monoclonal plasma cell disorder, and skin changes (POEMS)–associated multicentric CD (MCD) pathogenesis is driven by a monoclonal plasma cell population.
- Idiopathic MCD is poorly understood, although clinical data suggest a pathologic role for interleukin-6 in a subset of patients.

INTRODUCTION

Castleman disease (CD) describes a heterogeneous group of disorders defined by shared lymph node histopathological features, including atrophic or hyperplastic germinal centers, prominent follicular dendritic cells (FDCs), hypervascularization, polyclonal lymphoproliferation, and/or polytypic plasmacytosis.[1] Complicating diagnosis, these histopathologic features are not unique to CD but can be observed in other diseases as well.[2] Each subtype of CD has varying clinical features, causes, treatments, and outcomes. This article establishes the nomenclature required to discuss the different subtypes of CD (**Fig. 1**) and provides a summary of our current

Disclosure: D.C. Fajgenbaum receives research funding from Janssen Pharmaceuticals. D. Shilling has nothing to disclose.
Division of Translational Medicine and Human Genetics, Hospital of the University of Pennsylvania, 3400 Spruce Street, Silverstein 5, Suite S05094, Philadelphia, PA 19104, USA
* Corresponding author.
E-mail address: davidfa@pennmedicine.upenn.edu

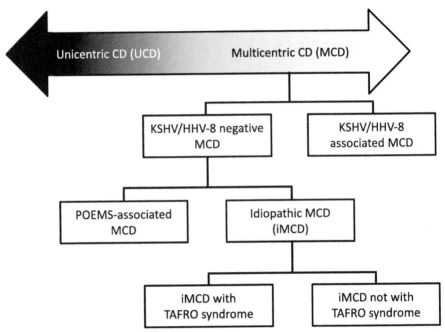

Fig. 1. CD classification. CD is classified based on the number of sites of enlarged lymph nodes with CD histopathological features. On one side of the CD spectrum is unicentric CD (UCD), solitary lymphadenopathy. On the other side of the spectrum is multicentric CD (MCD), multiple sites of lymphadenopathy. A hybrid of UCD and MCD, regionally restricted lymphadenopathy, has also been rarely observed. MCD is segmented based on Kaposi sarcoma-associated herpesvirus (KSHV)/human herpesvirus-8 (HHV-8) status. HHV-8–negative MCD is categorized as either polyneuropathy, organomegaly, endocrinopathy, monoclonal plasma cell disorder, and skin changes (POEMS)–associated or idiopathic MCD, the latter of which can be either with or without thrombocytopenia, anasarca, myelofibrosis, renal dysfunction, and organomegaly (TAFRO) syndrome.

understanding of the cause, cell types, signaling pathways, and effector cytokines implicated in pathogenesis.

CD is first classified based on the number of regions of enlarged lymph nodes that demonstrate histopathologic features consistent with CD. Unicentric CD (UCD) involves a single enlarged lymph node or region of lymph nodes, whereas multicentric CD (MCD) involves multiple regions of enlarged lymph nodes.

MCD is further divided based on Kaposi sarcoma-associated herpesvirus (KSHV)/ human herpesvirus-8 (HHV-8) infection status. In HHV-8–positive MCD, uncontrolled HHV-8 infection signals for excessive cytokine production, which causes the clinical and pathologic abnormalities.[3] Monoclonal plasma cells underlying coexisting polyneuropathy, organomegaly, endocrinopathy, monoclonal plasma cell disorder, and skin changes (POEMS) syndrome cause some cases (POEMS-associated MCD) of HHV-8–negative MCD, whereas others are idiopathic (iMCD). POEMS is a paraneoplastic syndrome that often co-occurs with MCD (POEMS-associated MCD).[4] iMCD is itself heterogeneous; recent work has identified at least one distinct clinical subtype of iMCD, which involves thrombocytopenia, anasarca, myelofibrosis, renal dysfunction, and organomegaly (TAFRO) syndrome (iMCD-TAFRO).[5]

UNICENTRIC CASTLEMAN DISEASE

Most patients with UCD do not experience systemic symptoms.[1] Typically, the enlarged lymph node will be discovered inadvertently, during care for another condition or because it is impeding on nearby organs. UCD is diagnosed by histopathologic examination of the excised lymph node. Removal of the node or region of nodes is almost always curative, but recurrences of UCD have been reported.[6] Thus, it is thought that the pathologic cell types and drivers are present in the excised lymph node. No cases of UCD have ever been reported to transition into MCD.

Cause

Viral, neoplastic, and reactive inflammatory mechanisms have all been proposed as etiologic mechanisms in UCD. Arguing against the viral hypothesis, T-Box Expressed in T cells, which is expressed by cells in the context of high interferon-γ during intracellular pathogen infection, was not found to be expressed by T or B cells in UCD lymph nodes.[7] In one study, all UCD lymph nodes were found to be Epstein-Barr virus (EBV) positive,[8] but this observation was not reproduced in a separate cohort.[9] Given the high prevalence of EBV infection and rarity of UCD, it is unlikely that EBV is a primary pathologic driver of UCD.

In contrast to the viral hypothesis, several lines of evidence suggest that UCD is most likely neoplastic. A study of lymphoproliferative disorders found that UCD lymph nodes have an increased number of small follicles with abnormally low proliferation, which is observed in follicular lymphoma so the investigators concluded this finding may be suggestive of neoplastic changes.[10] UCD is one of the most common causes of paraneoplastic pemphigus along with non-Hodgkin lymphoma and other hematologic neoplasia.[11] Cytogenetic anomalies have been reported in cultured lymph node stromal cells from several UCD cases.[12–15] In fact, one study identified modifications in chromosome segment 12q13 to 15, which is also commonly found in several benign mesenchymal tumors; another study identified a clonal cytogenetic anomaly (t[1;22] [p22;q13]) that was hypothesized to affect the megakaryoblastic leukemia 1 (MKL1) gene, which is implicated in acute megakaryocytic leukemia, and the endothelial cell growth factor 1 gene, which promotes angiogenesis and prevents cellular apoptosis. However, the most compelling evidence for the neoplastic hypothesis comes from a larger study that used conventional and methylation-specific polymerase chain reaction methods to assess monoclonality within UCD lymph node tissue. Monoclonality was detected in 19 of 25 UCD cases but not in 20 cases of lymphoid hyperplasia.[16] Rare reports of familial cases of UCD do exist, although genetic sequencing was not performed.[17,18]

Cell Type

The cell type responsible for driving UCD pathogenesis has not been definitively identified. However, the studies described earlier suggest the monoclonal cell harboring the genomic alterations may be stromal, specifically FDCs.[12,14–16] Consistent with these results, stromal cell overgrowth and FDC prominence and dysplasia are often seen in UCD.[19] FDCs are essential for germinal center formation and play a major role in directing lymphocytes into the appropriate regions within the lymph node and promoting B cell survival.[20] In further support of a role for neoplastic FDCs as a primary driver of UCD pathogenesis are reports of patients with UCD subsequently developing FDC sarcoma in the same region of lymph nodes.[21,22]

Signaling Pathways

Dysregulated signaling pathways have not been extensively studied in UCD. Cases describing overexpression of epidermal growth factor receptor[21] and interleukin

(IL)-6[23] may shed light on potential signaling pathways involved in other patients with UCD.

Effector Cytokines

In the small portion of UCD cases with systemic symptoms, IL-6 is likely to be the effector cytokine driving systemic symptoms.[24] However, IL-6 levels have not been systematically studied in several UCD cases and many cases do not have systemic symptoms. Interestingly, FDCs' role in orchestrating lymphocyte trafficking is largely mediated through the secretion of chemokine (C-X-C motif) ligand 13 (CXCL13) (also known as B lymphocyte chemoattractant), and dysplastic FDCs in UCD lymph nodes strongly express this chemokine.[22] Therefore, CXCL13 may play an important role in UCD; but again, CXCL13 levels have not been systematically studied in UCD.

Taken together, experimental data and pathologic characteristics suggest a clonal proliferation of FDCs as the etiologic driver and pathologic cell type in UCD. The authors propose that acquired mutations in these stromal cells result in UCD. Additional studies are needed to investigate this hypothesis.

HUMAN HERPESVIRUS-8–ASSOCIATED MULTICENTRIC CASTLEMAN DISEASE

Although lymph node histopathologic features overlap with those observed in UCD, MCD involves multiple regions of enlarged nodes. Patients with MCD also experience systemic symptoms, including progressive disease flares characterized by constitutional symptoms, cytopenias, hepatosplenomegaly, fluid accumulation, and cytokine storm–associated multiple organ system dysfunction. As detailed in the introduction of this article, MCD is categorized as either HHV-8–associated MCD, POEMS-associated MCD, or iMCD, each of which is discussed independently.

Cause

HHV-8 is the well-established etiologic cause of HHV-8–associated MCD.[25] Human immunodeficiency virus (HIV) infection or another cause of immunodeficiency enables HHV-8 to escape from host immune control, lytically replicate in lymph node plasmablasts, and signal for the release of cytokines that drive clinical and pathologic symptoms.[26,27]

Cell Type

HHV-8 infects B cells and plasmablasts, which can be detected by immunohistochemical staining of patients' lymph node for latency-associated nuclear antigen-1. Highlighting the critical role of B cells in HHV-8–associated MCD, their depletion with rituximab is a highly effective therapy.[28] Peripheral T cell levels, including polyfunctional effector memory CD8$^+$ T cells, have also been associated with HHV-8–associated MCD pathogenesis.[29]

Signaling Pathways

Researchers have found that upregulation of nuclear factor kappa-light-chain-enhancer of activated B cells (NF-κB) by latently expressed viral-FLICE (viral Fas-associating protein with death domain–like interleukin-1–converting enzyme) inhibitory protein or viral microRNA-K1 and upregulation of vascular endothelial growth factor (VEGF) and other factors by a viral G-protein couple receptor may be involved in HHV-8–associated MCD pathogenesis.[30] These secreted proteins induce B cell and plasma cell proliferation, angiogenesis, and an acute-phase reaction.[25]

Effector Cytokines

Human IL-6 and viral IL-6 (vIL-6) both play important roles in driving the B cell proliferation and symptoms observed in HHV-8–associated MCD. Mechanistically, vIL-6 can bind directly to the IL-6 receptor (gp130) and does not need its coreceptor, gp80, as human IL-6 does.[30] Therefore, it is possible that a wider range of cells may be affected by vIL-6 than human IL-6.

HUMAN HERPESVIRUS-8–NEGATIVE MULTICENTRIC CASTLEMAN DISEASE

When HHV-8 infection was first associated with MCD in 1994, the CD research community almost entirely shifted its focus to studying HHV-8–associated MCD. Until recently, there was little recognition that a large proportion of patients with MCD are HHV-8 negative. Despite having a similar incidence to HHV-8–associated MCD,[31] HHV-8–negative MCD has received a fraction of the research attention and is significantly less well understood. The following discussion presents our current molecular and etiologic understanding of HHV-8–negative MCD, which is subclassified into POEMS-associated MCD and iMCD.

POEMS–Associated Multicentric Castleman Disease

Cause/cell type

POEMS-associated MCD is thought to be caused by cytokine production from monoclonal plasma cells that have undergone genomic events, such as translocations or deletions. Nearly all POEMS cases are λ light chain restricted.[4] Highlighting the primary role of the monoclonal plasma cell population in POEMS pathogenesis, radiation to an isolated plasmacytoma is often curative.[4]

Signaling pathways/effector cytokines

VEGF is the cytokine that best correlates with disease activity,[32] although other cytokines must also contribute because VEGF blockade has provided only mixed results clinically.[33] Other cytokines proposed to drive POEMS symptoms are IL-6, IL-12, transforming growth factor–1β, and tumor necrosis factor–α.[34]

Idiopathic Multicentric Castleman Disease

Cause

The cause of iMCD is unknown. The heterogeneity of the disease and overlapping clinical and pathologic abnormalities with other immunologic disorders suggest that multiple processes each involving immune dysregulation and a common pathway of increased cytokines may give rise to iMCD in different subsets of patients.[35] In fact, recent work has identified 2 subgroups of patients with iMCD, iMCD-TAFRO and iMCD–non-TAFRO, which may represent different causes. To promote research aimed at uncovering the cause of iMCD, the CD research community, led by the Castleman Disease Collaborative Network (CDCN), recently hypothesized 4 candidate etiologically drivers of iMCD pathogenesis (**Fig. 2**), which are described later.

Autoimmune

iMCD may be due to self-reactive antibodies, which stimulate the release of cytokines. Autoimmune diseases can demonstrate clinical and histopathologic features that are identical to iMCD. Nearly all lymph nodes of patients with rheumatoid arthritis and 15% to 30% of lymph nodes from patients with systemic lupus erythematosus display CD histopathologic features.[36,37] Patients with iMCD respond to therapies used to treat autoimmune disease, such as anti–IL-6 receptor therapy and cyclosporine.[38] Approximately 30% of iMCD case reports found autoantibodies and autoimmunity.[31]

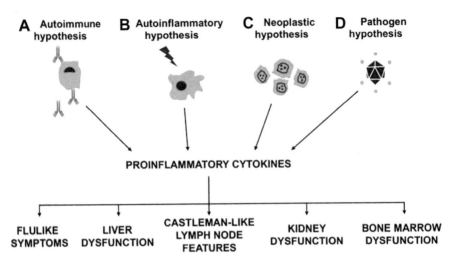

Fig. 2. Hypothesized etiologic drivers of iMCD. The CD research community, led by the CDCN, recently proposed 4 candidate etiologic drivers of iMCD pathogenesis: iMCD may be due to (*A*) self-reactive antibodies, (*B*) germline mutations in genes regulating inflammation, (*C*) acquired oncogenic mutations, or (*D*) an infection with a pathogen. (*Adapted from* Supplement to: Fajgenbaum DC, Ruth JR, Kelleher D, et al. The collaborative network approach: a new framework to accelerate Castleman's disease and other rare disease research. Lancet Haematol 2016;3(4):e150–2; with permission.)

However, it is unclear if these autoantibodies are etiologically responsible for iMCD, propagators of inflammation, or secondary to a primary disease driver.

Autoinflammatory iMCD may be due to germline mutations in genes regulating inflammation. A germline mutation in the Mediterranean fever gene, often found in familial Mediterranean fever (FMF) syndrome, was described in a reported iMCD case.[39] Whether this is a novel genetic cause of iMCD or an atypical case of FMF is unclear. A child with a multicentric Castleman-like syndrome was found to have homozygous mutations in cat eye syndrome critical region protein 1, which encodes adenosine deaminase 2 (ADA2).[40] Deficiency of ADA2 is known to stimulate IL-6 induction through adenosine A2B receptor activation.[41] An increased proportion of patients with iMCD harbored a polymorphism in the IL-6 receptor (IL-6R) gene compared with healthy controls in a recent study. Individuals with this polymorphism expressed significantly higher levels of soluble IL-6R, which can contribute to increased IL-6 activity through the trans-signaling pathway.[42] Although interesting, these associations require confirmation and functional analysis.

Neoplastic iMCD may be due to acquired oncogenic mutations. iMCD clinical and histopathologic features overlap with those of lymphoma, and patients with iMCD have an increased rate of malignancy compared with age-matched controls.[31] Interestingly, in a small study of 4 iMCD cases, all were found to have monoclonality in the lymph node.[16] The monoclonal cells were most likely stromal, as the lymphocytes in those cases were polyclonal and lymphocytes in other MCD cases are typically polyclonal.[43] A patient with HIV-negative MCD, who was not tested for HHV-8, was found to have a somatic translocation (46,XY,t[7;14] [p22;q22]) in lymph node tissue at the IL-6 locus (7p21–22).[44]

Pathogen iMCD may be due to an infection. Patients with HHV-8–negative MCD share clinicopathologic features with HHV-8–associated MCD, but a pathogen-driver has not been discovered to date. Thus, the authors hypothesized that a pathogen, possibly a virus with homology to HHV-8, could be driving iMCD pathogenesis. EBV, HHV-6, hepatitis B virus, cytomegalovirus, toxoplasma, and mycobacterium tuberculosis infection have all been reported in at least one case of iMCD.[8,45–49] Whether these infections are pathologic, coincidental, or secondary to iMCD immune dysfunction remains to be determined.

Cell type The limited research conducted to date has generated conflicting reports regarding the cell type responsible for driving iMCD pathogenesis and/or producing IL-6. Candidate cell types include lymphocytes, plasma cells, monocytes, endothelial cells, and FDCs.[23,50–53] Despite the lack of consistent reports, some evidence for a pathogenic role of B cells in some cases does exist. CD5$^+$ mantle zone B cells in HIV-negative (HHV-8-unknown) MCD cases proliferate and secrete autoantibodies because of factors produced by fibroblastic reticular dendritic cells.[19] A subset of patients with iMCD respond clinically to B cell depletion with rituximab, supporting B cells as a potential driver or important contributor in some iMCD cases.[31] However, it is clear that other cell types are involved in iMCD pathogenesis because B cell depletion is not effective in all patients.[31] Elevated serum soluble IL-2 receptor, a marker of T cell activation, was found in 20 of 21 published cases of iMCD, suggesting a potential role of T cells in iMCD pathogenesis.[31]

Signaling pathways/effector cytokines Although the pathologic cell types in iMCD are unknown, it is clear from human and animal studies that IL-6 is sufficient and, in a subset of patients, necessary to drive iMCD symptomatology, histopathology, and pathogenesis. IL-6 is a pleiotropic cytokine involved in the induction of a wide range of activities, including plasmacytosis, hypergammaglobulinemia, thrombocytosis, acute-phase protein production by the liver, and activation of macrophages and T cells.[25] Elevated IL-6 was first associated with iMCD in 1989.[52] Clinical symptoms often wax and wane with IL-6 levels, which can be highly elevated in patients with iMCD during disease flare.[54] Mouse models of excess IL-6 production recapitulated many features of human iMCD, and the administration of anti–IL-6R monoclonal antibody (mAb) is effective in treating such mice.[55,56] Moreover, the administration of recombinant IL-6 to humans can lead to an iMCD-like syndrome.[57] Interruption of IL-6 signaling with anti–IL-6 or anti–IL-6R mAb is effective at ameliorating symptoms and shrinking lymph nodes in some patients.[31] Siltuximab, an anti–IL-6 mAb, became the first, and is currently the only, Food and Drug Administration–approved therapy for iMCD based on improved clinical symptoms and lymph node size in 34% of patients compared with 0% for placebo in a double-blind phase II clinical trial.[58] However, 66% of patients in the clinical trial did not respond to siltuximab treatment, approximately half of which did not have elevated IL-6 levels.[59] It is, therefore, likely that other cytokines or soluble factors can also drive iMCD pathogenesis. Considering the redundancy of functions played by cytokines, it is certainly plausible that the hypersecretion of similar cytokines could result in a related clinical phenotype.

Evidence has been slowly accumulating for a role of additional cytokines in iMCD pathogenesis. A systematic review of iMCD case reports found that VEGF was elevated in 16 of 20 cases,[31] a finding that was subsequently confirmed in 17 cases.[60] Elevated VEGF levels may explain the capillary leak syndrome and eruptive cherry hemangiomatosis observed in some iMCD cases.[61] Mechanistic target of rapamycin (mTOR), which regulates VEGF expression, has also been implicated, as a relapsed/refractory iMCD-TAFRO case experienced a prolonged remission on the mTOR inhibitor sirolimus.[5] IL-1β has also been proposed as a possible driver of iMCD pathogenesis. Administration of anti–IL-1 therapy has been reported to be effective in a few case reports, including 2 patients with iMCD refractory to anti–IL-6 therapy.[62,63] IL-1β is upstream of IL-6 and VEGF in the proinflammatory cascade and leads to IL-6 production through NF-κB activation. Regardless of cause, excessive activation of inflammatory pathways in immune cells leads to histopathologic changes in the lymph node and systemic symptoms observed in iMCD.

FUTURE DIRECTIONS

This article presents our current understanding of the pathogenesis for each subtype of CD as of 2017. Although our understanding of CD has slowly improved over the last 6 decades, leading to improved patient survival and quality of life, additional research is needed. The authors anticipate significant progress to be made in the coming years through research studies led by the CDCN, including the ACCELERATE (Advancing Castleman Care with an Electronic Longitudinal registry, E-Repository, And Treatment/Effectiveness research) Natural History Registry (www.CDCN.org/ACCELERATE), which is open for patient self-enrollment.

REFERENCES

1. Waterston A, Bower M. Fifty years of multicentric Castleman's disease. Acta Oncol 2004;43(8):698–704.
2. Fajgenbaum DC, Uldrick TS, Bagg A, et al. International, evidence-based consensus diagnostic criteria for HHV-8–negative/idiopathic multicentric Castleman disease. Blood 2017;129(12):1646–57.
3. Oksenhendler E, Duarte M, Soulier J, et al. Multicentric Castleman's disease in HIV infection: a clinical and pathological study of 20 patients. AIDS 1996;10(1):61–7.
4. Dispenzieri A. POEMS syndrome and Castleman's disease. In: Zimmerman TM, Kumar SK, editors. Biology and management of unusual plasma cell dyscrasias. New York: Springer; 2017. p. 41–69.
5. Iwaki N, Fajgenbaum DC, Nabel CS, et al. Clinicopathologic analysis of TAFRO syndrome demonstrates a distinct subtype of HHV-8-negative multicentric Castleman disease. Am J Hematol 2016;91(2):220–6.
6. Talat N, Schulte KM. Castleman's disease: systematic analysis of 416 patients from the literature. Oncologist 2011;16(9):1316–24.
7. Johrens K, Anagnostopoulos I, Durkop H, et al. Different T-bet expression patterns characterize particular reactive lymphoid tissue lesions. Histopathology 2006;48(4):343–52.
8. Chen CH, Liu HC, Hung TT, et al. Possible roles of Epstein-Barr virus in Castleman disease. J Cardiothorac Surg 2009;4:31.
9. Al-Maghrabi JA, Kamel-Reid S, Bailey DJ. Lack of evidence of Epstein-Barr virus infection in patients with Castleman's disease. Molecular genetic analysis. Neurosciences (Riyadh) 2006;11(4):279–83.
10. Bryant RJ. Ki67 staining pattern as a diagnostic tool in the evaluation of lymphoproliferative disorders. Histopathology 2006;48(5):505–15.
11. Lehman VT, Barrick BJ, Pittelkow MR, et al. Diagnostic imaging in paraneoplastic autoimmune multiorgan syndrome: retrospective single site study and literature review of 225 patients. Int J Dermatol 2015;54(4):424–37.
12. Chen WC, Jones D, Ho CL, et al. Cytogenetic anomalies in hyaline vascular Castleman disease: report of two cases with reappraisal of histogenesis. Cancer Genet Cytogenet 2006;164(2):110–7.

13. Cokelaere KK. Hyaline vascular Castleman's disease with HMGIC rearrangement in follicular dendritic cells: molecular evidence of mesenchymal tumorigenesis. Am J Surg Pathol 2002;26(5):662–9.

14. Pauwels P, Dal Cin P, Vlasveld LT, et al. A chromosomal abnormality in hyaline vascular Castleman's disease: evidence for clonal proliferation of dysplastic stromal cells. Am J Surg Pathol 2000;24(6):882–8.

15. Reichard KK, Robinett S, Foucar MK. Clonal cytogenetic abnormalities in the plasma cell variant of Castleman disease. Cancer Genet 2011;204(6):323–7.

16. Chang KC, Wang YC, Hung LY, et al. Monoclonality and cytogenetic abnormalities in hyaline vascular Castleman disease. Mod Pathol 2013;27(6):823–31.

17. Leslie C, Shingde M, Kwok F, et al. T-lymphoblastic proliferation and florid multifocal follicular dendritic cell proliferation occurring in hyaline-vascular Castleman disease in a patient with a possible familial predisposition. J Hematop 2013;6(4): 237–44.

18. Martin CC. Castleman's disease in identical twins. Virchows Arch A Pathol Anat Histol 1982;395(1):77–85.

19. Menke DM, Tiemann M, Camoriano JK, et al. Diagnosis of Castleman's disease by identification of an immunophenotypically aberrant population of mantle zone B lymphocytes in paraffin-embedded lymph node biopsies. Am J Clin Pathol 1996;105(3):268–76.

20. Aguzzi A, Kranich J, Krautler NJ. Follicular dendritic cells: origin, phenotype, and function in health and disease. Trends Immunol 2014;35(3):105–13.

21. Sun X, Chang KC, Abruzzo LV, et al. Epidermal growth factor receptor expression in follicular dendritic cells: a shared feature of follicular dendritic cell sarcoma and Castleman's disease. Hum Pathol 2003;34(9):835–40.

22. Vermi WW. Identification of CXCL13 as a new marker for follicular dendritic cell sarcoma. J Pathol 2008;216(3):356–64.

23. Post GR. Diagnostic utility of interleukin-6 expression by immunohistochemistry in differentiating Castleman disease subtypes and reactive lymphadenopathies. Ann Clin Lab Sci 2016;46(5):474–9.

24. Vinzio S, Ciarloni L, Schlienger JL, et al. Isolated microcytic anemia disclosing a unicentric Castleman disease: the interleukin-6/hepcidin pathway? Eur J Intern Med 2008;19(5):367–9.

25. Kishimoto T. IL-6: from its discovery to clinical applications. Int Immunol 2010; 22(5):347–52.

26. Dossier A, Meignin V, Fieschi C, et al. Human herpesvirus 8-related Castleman disease in the absence of HIV infection. Clin Infect Dis 2013;56(6):833–42.

27. Suda T, Katano H, Delsol G, et al. HHV-8 infection status of AIDS-unrelated and AIDS-associated multicentric Castleman's disease. Pathol Int 2001;51:671–9.

28. Bower M, Newsom-Davis T, Naresh K, et al. Clinical features and outcome in HIV-associated multicentric Castleman's disease. J Clin Oncol 2011;29(18):2481–6.

29. Guihot A, Oksenhendler E, Galicier L, et al. Multicentric Castleman disease is associated with polyfunctional effector memory HHV-8-specific CD8 T cells. Blood 2008;111(3):1387–95.

30. Uldrick TS, Polizzotto MN, Yarchoan R. Recent advances in Kaposi sarcoma herpesvirus-associated multicentric Castleman disease. Curr Opin Oncol 2012; 24(5):495–505.

31. Liu AY, Nabel CS, Finkelman BS, et al. Idiopathic multicentric Castleman's disease: a systematic literature review. Lancet Haematol 2016;3(4):e163–75.

32. D'Souza AA. The utility of plasma vascular endothelial growth factor levels in the diagnosis and follow-up of patients with POEMS syndrome. Blood 2001;118(17): 4663–5.
33. Sekiguchi YY. Ambiguous effects of anti-VEGF monoclonal antibody (bevacizumab) for POEMS syndrome. J Neurol Neurosurg Psychiatry 2013;84(12):1346–8.
34. Warsame RR. POEMS syndrome: an enigma. Curr Hematol Malig Rep 2017; 12(2):85–95.
35. Fajgenbaum DC, van Rhee F, Nabel CS. HHV-8-negative, idiopathic multicentric Castleman disease: novel insights into biology, pathogenesis, and therapy. Blood 2014;123(19):2924–33.
36. Kojima M, Motoori T, Asano S, et al. Histological diversity of reactive and atypical proliferative lymph node lesions in systemic lupus erythematosus patients. Pathol Res Pract 2007;203(6):423–31.
37. Kojima M, Motoori T, Nakamura S. Benign, atypical and malignant lymphoproliferative disorders in rheumatoid arthritis patients. Biomed Pharmacother 2006; 60(10):663–72.
38. Kawabata H, Kadowaki N, Nishikori M, et al. Clinical features and treatment of multicentric Castleman's disease : a retrospective study of 21 Japanese patients at a single institute. J Clin Exp Hematop 2013;53(1):69–77.
39. Kone-Paut I, Hentgen V, Guillaume-Czitrom S, et al. The clinical spectrum of 94 patients carrying a single mutated MEFV allele. Rheumatology (Oxford) 2009; 48(7):840–2.
40. Van Eyck LL. Mutant ADA2 in vasculopathies. N Engl J Med 2014;371(5):478–9.
41. Dai Y, Zhang W, Wen J, et al. A(2B) adenosine receptor–mediated induction of IL-6 promotes CKD. J Am Soc Nephrol 2011;22(5):890–901.
42. Stone K, Woods E, Szmania SM, et al. Interleukin-6 receptor polymorphism is prevalent in HIV-negative Castleman disease and is associated with increased soluble interleukin-6 receptor levels. PLoS One 2013;8(1):e54610.
43. Al-Maghrabi J, Kamel-Reid S, Bailey D. Immunoglobulin and T-cell receptor gene rearrangement in Castleman's disease: molecular genetic analysis. Histopathology 2006;48(3):233–8.
44. Nakamura H, Nakaseko C, Ishii A, et al. Chromosomal abnormalities in Castleman's disease with high levels of serum interleukin-6. Rinsho Ketsueki 1993; 34(2):212–7 [in Japanese].
45. Barozzi P, Luppi M, Masini L, et al. Lymphotropic herpes virus (EBV, HHV-6, HHV-8) DNA sequences in HIV negative Castleman's disease. Clin Mol Pathol 1996; 49(4):M232–5.
46. Bowne WB, Lewis JJ, Filippa DA, et al. The management of unicentric and multicentric Castleman's disease: a report of 16 cases and a review of the literature. Cancer 1999;85(3):706–17.
47. Jones EL, Crocker J, Gregory J, et al. Angiofollicular lymph node hyperplasia (Castleman's disease): an immunohistochemical and enzyme-histochemical study of the hyaline-vascular form of lesion. J Pathol 1984;144(2):131–47.
48. Murray PG, Deacon E, Young LS, et al. Localization of Epstein-Barr virus in Castleman's disease by in situ hybridization and immunohistochemistry. Hematol Pathol 1995;9(1):17–26.
49. Yuan XG, Chen FF, Zhu YM, et al. High prevalence of hepatitis B virus infection in HIV-negative Castleman's disease. Ann Hematol 2012;91(6):857–61.
50. Lai YM, Li M, Liu CL, et al. Expression of interleukin-6 and its clinicopathological significance in Castleman's disease. Zhonghua Xue Ye Xue Za Zhi 2013;34(5): 404–8 [in Chinese].

51. Leger-Ravet MB, Peuchmaur M, Devergne O, et al. Interleukin-6 gene expression in Castleman's disease. Blood 1991;78(11):2923–30.
52. Yoshizaki K, Matsuda T, Nishimoto N, et al. Pathogenic significance of interleukin-6 (IL-6/BSF-2) in Castleman's disease. Blood 1989;74(4):1360–7.
53. Yu L, Tu M, Cortes J, et al. Clinical and pathological characteristics of HIV- and HHV-8–negative Castleman disease. Blood 2017;129(12):1658–68.
54. van Rhee F, Stone K, Szmania S, et al. Castleman disease in the 21st century: an update on diagnosis, assessment, and therapy. Clin Adv Hematol Oncol 2010; 8(7):486–98.
55. Alonzi T, Gorgoni B, Screpanti I, et al. Interleukin-6 and CAAT/enhancer binding protein beta-deficient mice act as tools to dissect the IL-6 signalling pathway and IL-6 regulation. Immunobiology 1997;198(1–3):144–56.
56. Brandt SJ, Bodine DM, Dunbar CE, et al. Dysregulated interleukin 6 expression produces a syndrome resembling Castleman's disease in mice. J Clin Invest 1990;86(2):592–9.
57. van Gameren MM, Willemse PH, Mulder NH, et al. Effects of recombinant human interleukin-6 in cancer patients: a phase I-II study. Blood 1994;84(5):1434–41.
58. van Rhee F, Wong RS, Munshi N, et al. Siltuximab for multicentric Castleman's disease: a randomised, double-blind, placebo-controlled trial. Lancet Oncol 2014;15(9):966–74.
59. Casper C, Chaturvedi S, Munshi N, et al. Analysis of inflammatory and anemia-related biomarkers in a randomized, double-blind, placebo-controlled study of siltuximab (anti-IL6 monoclonal antibody) in patients with multicentric Castleman disease. Clin Cancer Res 2015;21(19):4294–304.
60. Iwaki N, Gion Y, Kondo E, et al. Elevated serum interferon γ-induced protein 10 kDa is associated with TAFRO syndrome. Sci Rep 2017;7:42316.
61. Fajgenbaum D, Rosenbach M, van Rhee F, et al. Eruptive cherry hemangiomatosis associated with multicentric Castleman disease: a case report and diagnostic clue. JAMA Dermatol 2013;149(2):204–8.
62. El-Osta H, Janku F, Kurzrock R. Successful treatment of Castleman's disease with interleukin-1 receptor antagonist (anakinra). Mol Cancer Ther 2010;9(6):1485–8.
63. Galeotti C, Tran TA, Franchi-Abella S, et al. IL-1RA agonist (anakinra) in the treatment of multifocal Castleman disease: case report. J Pediatr Hematol Oncol 2008;30(12):920–4.

The Role of Interleukin-6 in Castleman Disease

Kazuyuki Yoshizaki, MD, PhD[a],*, Shinichi Murayama, PhD[a], Hiroki Ito[a],
Tomohiro Koga, MD, PhD[b,c]

KEYWORDS

- Interleukin-6 • Humanized anti-IL-6 receptor antibody • Tocilizumab
- Chimeric anti-IL-6 antibody • Siltuximab • Multicentric Castleman disease
- IL-6 blocking therapy

KEY POINTS

- Since its discovery in 1956, Castleman disease has been the target of ongoing research, which has led to safe and effective treatment.
- Interleukin-6 (IL-6) has been implicated in Castleman disease. Most systemic symptoms of plasma cell variant of Castleman disease were linked to the hyperfunction of IL-6, which is continuously produced in the affected lymph node in 1989.
- A humanized anti-IL-6 receptor antibody (myeloma receptor antibody [MRA], tocilizumab, actemra) was generated in 1993 and used in the treatment of multicentric Castleman disease (MCD).
- Most MCD symptoms and abnormal laboratory findings were reported to be improved by tocilizumab and siltuximab therapy, respectively, in 2000 and 2009.
- Although other treatment agents for MCD are being refined, such as JAK inhibitors and rapamycin, current research is now focused on discovering the mechanisms that render tocilizumab effective in treating MCD.

INTRODUCTION

Castleman disease is a lymphoproliferative disease with benign hyperplastic lymph nodes and is classified pathologically in 2 forms: hyaline vascular and plasma cell. Multicentric Castleman disease (MCD) has the characteristics of plasma cell infiltration in the

Disclosure Statement: K. Yoshizaki disclosed grants from the Ministry of Health, Labor and Welfare Japan (H27-Nanchi-002). K. Yoshizaki has a patent royalty from Chugai Pharmaceutical. S. Murayama and T. Koga have no conflict of interest.
[a] Department of Biomolecular Science and Regulation, The Institute of Scientific and Industrial Research, Osaka University, 8-1 Mihogaoka, Ibaraki, Osaka 567-0047, Japan; [b] Department of Immunology and Rheumatology, Division of Advanced Preventive Medical Sciences, Nagasaki University Graduate School of Biomedical Sciences, 1-12-4 Sakamoto, Nagasaki 852-8523, Japan; [c] Center for Bioinformatics and Molecular Medicine, Nagasaki University Graduate School of Biomedical Sciences, 1-12-4 Sakamoto, Nagasaki 852-8523, Japan
* Corresponding author.
E-mail address: kyoshi@sanken.osaka-u.ac.jp

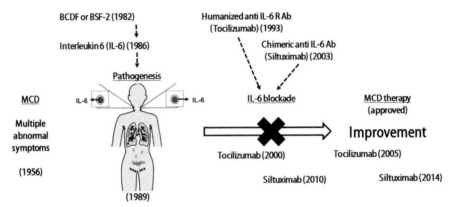

Fig. 1. Development of IL-6 blocking therapy on MCD. Ab, antibody.

affected lymph nodes with systemic manifestations, such as fever, fatigue, anemia, hypergammaglobulinemia, hypoalbuminemia, and an increase in acute phase proteins, such as C-reactive protein (CRP), serum amyloid A (SAA), fibrinogen, and hepcidin. Interleukin-6 (IL-6) is a pleiotropic cytokine that regulates immune responses, induces acute phase proteins, and supports hematopoiesis. IL-6 has been implicated in Castleman disease, and over the years, there has been an increasing body of research that aims to uncover the role IL-6 as well as its mechanism of action in Castleman disease.

This article is a review of IL-6 and IL-6 blocking therapy for MCD (**Fig. 1**). The authors describe how IL-6 was first identified and how anti-IL-6 treatments have progressed over the years, and discuss discoveries that have been made about the mechanism whereby IL-6 blocking agents alleviate MCD. This report discusses the case of 2 patients with plasma cell variant Castleman disease that allowed the first confirmation of IL-6 production in their affected lymph nodes. These 2 cases highlighted the correlation between IL-6 serum levels and clinical features, indicating that dysregulated production of IL-6 in enlarged lymph nodes might be responsible for the systemic manifestations of MCD. In later studies, attempts have been made to treat MCD using IL-6 blocking therapy with a humanized anti-IL-6 receptor antibody (tocilizumab) or a chimeric anti-IL-6 antibody (siltuximab). Results from these studies have demonstrated that both forms of IL-6 blocking therapy are safe and have delivered remarkable results in treating MCD patients.

DISCOVERY, PRODUCTION, AND FUNCTION OF INTERLEUKIN-6

IL-6 was first isolated from lymphocyte culture supernatants and was originally characterized and cloned as a B-cell differentiation factor (BCDF or BSF-2) that induces the final maturation of B cells into immunoglobulin-producing cells.[1,2] IL-6 is a glycoprotein secreted by T cells, B cells, and macrophages and has an apparent molecular weight of 22 to 27 kDa. It is composed of 212 amino-acid residues, including 28 amino-acids signal peptides (**Fig. 2**A).[3] IL-6 is produced by various cells, including immunocompetent cells (T cell, B cell, macrophage, dendritic cells), hematopoietic cells, endothelial cells, epithelial cells, fibroblasts, synovial cells, and osteoblasts. IL-6 production is induced through innate and acquired immune responses and is augmented in response to various antigenic stimulations, including bacteria, virus, several biomolecules, cytokines, and chemokines. IL-6 has pleiotropic functions, as shown in **Fig. 3**. IL-6 induces cell growth and differentiation, cytokines, immunoglobulins, and acute phase proteins[4–6] as well as the activation of sympathetic nerve, including the central nervous system. Therefore, when IL-6 production increases or

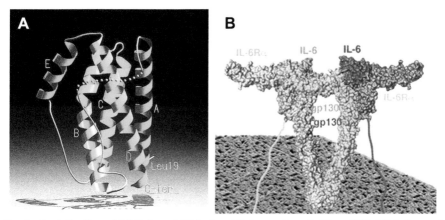

Fig. 2. Crystalization of (*A*) IL-6, and (*B*) IL-6 and IL-6 receptors (IL-6R, gp130). (*A*) IL-6 crystal structure. (*B*) IL-6/IL-6R/gp130 complex (hexamer). IL-6 binds to IL-6R and then to gp130; this IL-6/IL-6R/gp130 complex transduced IL-6 signal into the cell through gp130. ([*A*] *From* Somers W, Stahl M, Seehra JS. 1.9 Å crystal structure of interleukin 6: implications for a novel mode of receptor dimerization and signaling. EMBO J 1997;16(5):990, with permission; and [*B*] *Modified from* Skiniotis G, Lupardus PJ, Martick M, et al. Structural organization of a full-length gp130/LIF-R cytokine receptor transmembrane complex. Mol Cell 2008;31(5):744, with permission.)

IL-6 function is augmented in vivo, various symptoms, such as fatigue, low appetite, weight loss, high fever, and lymph node swelling, as well as abnormal laboratory findings such as renal dysfunction, anemia, osteoporosis, thrombocytosis, hypoalbuminemia, increase of acute phase proteins (CRP, SAA, fibrinogen, hepcidin, and so forth), and increase of polyclonal immunoglobulins occur (see **Fig. 3**).

INTERLEUKIN-6 RECEPTOR SYSTEM AND SIGNAL TRANSDUCTION PATHWAY

IL-6 signaling is mediated by 2 unique cell surface receptor molecules: the IL-6 receptor (IL-6R), a binding molecule, and the signal-transducing receptor glycoprotein, gp130, which binds the IL-6/IL-6R complex. IL-6 signaling is transduced into cells by 2 pathways, one is via membrane-bound IL-6 (mIL-6R) complexed with gp130, with which IL-6 forms a hexamer consisting of a pair of IL-6/mIL-6R/gp130 complex (**Fig. 2**B). IL-6R also exists as soluble IL-6R (sIL-6R), which mediates the transsignal pathway via a hexamer formed by a pair of IL-6/sIL-6R/gp130 complex.[7] Therefore, sIL-6 is an agonist of IL-6 signaling that increases in inflammatory states; on the other hand, soluble gp130 (sgp130) is an antagonist of IL-6 signaling and prevents IL-6/sIL-6R complex from binding to membrane-bound gp130. Therefore, sgp130 may be a natural IL-6 inhibitor or a brake in vivo. The mechanism of intracellular signaling of the IL-6 receptor system is shown in **Fig. 4**A.

REVELATION OF THE ROLE OF INTERLEUKIN-6 IN THE PATHOGENESIS OF CASTLEMAN DISEASE

In 1956, Benjamin Castleman and colleagues[8] reported a group of patients with localized benign hyperplastic mediastinal lymph node characterized by hyperplasia of lymphoid follicles and capillary proliferation with endothelial hyperplasia, resembling thymoma. Subsequently, in 1985, Frizzera and colleagues[9] classified Castleman disease into 2 histopathologic types: hyaline-vascular and plasma cell infiltration. The latter form of the disease is accompanied by multiple systemic manifestations, including general fatigue,

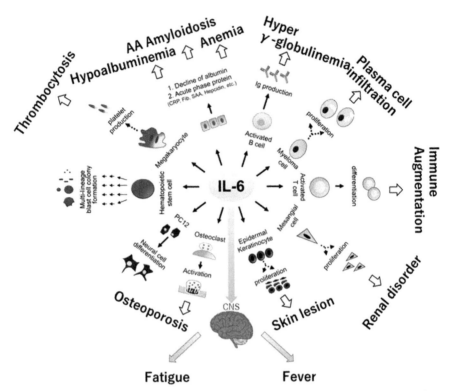

Fig. 3. IL-6 functions in vitro, abnormal findings. Symptoms may be linked to the overfunction of IL-6 in vivo. IL-6 shows multiple functions through multitargeted cells. IL-6 activation induces the multiple symptoms in vivo. CNS, central nervous system; Fib, fibrinogen PC 12, name of cell line.

fever, anemia, polyclonal hypergammaglobulinemia, and hypoalbuminemia, and occasionally, is associated with pulmonary disease and renal dysfunction.

In 1986, the authors examined 2 patients with plasma cell variant Castleman disease characterized by multiple clinical manifestations. Patient 1 was a 14-year-old

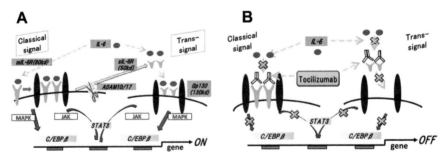

Fig. 4. IL-6 signal pathway and the mode of action of anti-IL-6R antibody. (*A*) IL-6, IL-6 receptor system and soluble form of IL-6R and gp130 contribute to IL-6 signals on the cell surface via a classical pathway with membrane IL-6R, and a transsignal pathway with sIL-6R. (*B*) Inhibition of IL-6 signal by a humanized anti-IL-6R antibody (MRA, tocilizumab, actemra). Tocilizumab inhibits IL-6 binding on mIL-6R in the classical pathway and on sIL-6R in the transsignal pathway.

Table 1
Clinical and laboratory findings before and after resection of a hyperplastic lymph node

Patient (Age, Sex)	Before and After Surgery	Affected Lymph Nodes	Clinical Symptoms	Hb (g/dL)	ESR (mm/h)	IgG (mg/dL)	IgA (mg/dL)	Immunoglobulins IgM (mg/dL)	IgE (U/mL)	CRP (mg/dL)	IL-6 (pg/mL)
1 (14, F)	Before	Solitary	(+)	9.1	157	4350	468	332	12	20.70	110
	After (2 wk)	No	(−)	11.6	22	2471	190	253	9	0.05	ND
	After (4 mo)	No	(−)	12.9	6	1813	165	246	ND	0.04	30
2 (52, F)	Before	Multiple	(+)	10.1	138	4650	1040	180	19,900	5.80	70
	After (1 mo)	Multiple	(+)	9.0	144	5320	941	179	ND	5.70	ND
	After (4 mo)	Multiple	(+)	8.2	144	4280	832	163	13,200	12.40	68

Clinical symptoms of 2 patients showed fatigue, fever, and arthritis. P1 had a solitary large lymph node at mediastinum. P2 had a large lymph node in abnormal cavity with enlarged lymph nodes at neck, axillary, and inguinal.

Abbreviations: ESR, erythrocyte sedimentation rate; ND, not done.

Modified from Yoshizaki K, Matsuda T, Nishimoto N, et al. Pathogenic significance of interleukin 6 (IL-6/BSF-2) in Castleman's disease. Blood 1989;74(4):1360; with permission.

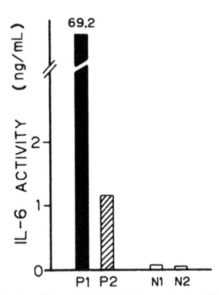

Fig. 5. IL-6 production by the affected lymph nodes in patients with MCD. IL-6 activity in the culture supernatants from the lymph nodes of 2 patients: P1 (*black bar*) and P2 (*shaded bar*) produced high levels; on the contrary, lower levels were observed in the control group (N1, N2: *white bars*). (*Modified from* Yoshizaki K, Matsuda T, Nishimoto N, et al. Pathogenic significance of interleukin 6 (IL-6/BSF-2) in Castleman's disease. Blood 1989;74(4):1361; with permission.)

girl with only a localized enlarged lymph node at mediastinum, thus having unicentric Castleman disease. Patient 2, a 52-year-old woman, had enlarged multicentric lymph nodes swollen at the neck, axillary, inguinal, and also a large lymph node in abdominal cavity at para-aortic region.[10]

As summarized in **Table 1**, after resecting the enlarged lymph node from each patient, all abnormal findings in patient 1 disappeared and her test results returned to normal with a marked reduction in serum IL-6 levels. On the other hand, in patient 2, symptoms and abnormal laboratory findings, such as elevated serum IL-6 levels, persisted after surgical removal of the enlarged abdominal hyperplastic lymph node.

To confirm the production of IL-6 in the affected lymph nodes, IL-6 was quantified in the culture supernatants of lymph node blocks taken from each of the 2 patients. IL-6 was also quantified in swollen lymph node blocks taken from noninflammatory controls. IL-6 levels in the culture supernatants were elevated in both patients compared with the controls (**Fig. 5**). Immunohistochemical analysis using an anti-IL-6 antibody confirmed the presence of IL-6 in the germinal center of the affected lymph nodes. This clinical and laboratory evidence suggested that IL-6 production in the germinal center of hyperplastic lymph nodes was a key factor instrumental to causing the array of clinical manifestations in Castleman disease.

BLOCKING INTERLEUKIN-6 FUNCTION WITH A HUMANIZED ANTI-INTERLEUKIN-6 RECEPTOR ANTIBODY

If continuous production of IL-6 is a key pathogenetic factor of plasma cell variant Castleman disease, then it seemed logical to reason that administering an IL-6 blocking treatment may alleviate the patients' symptoms. There are several methods for blocking IL-6: inhibiting IL-6 production, IL-6 binding on IL-6 receptor, and interrupting intracellular signaling.

Although the authors first tried to obtain antibodies against human IL-6, they could not generate such antibodies in hybridoma cells, because IL-6 is a hybridoma growth factor. Kishimoto and colleagues[11] generated a mouse anti-human IL-6R antibody in a B-cell hybrid cell line hybridized with spleen cells from a mouse immunized with sIL-6R. The mouse anti-human IL-6R antibody was engineered to be humanized, and the recombinant humanized antibody was conveniently produced in a hamster cell line. This humanized anti-human IL-6R antibody (investigational product code: myeloma receptor antibody [MRA]) was later shown to have little antigenicity in humans and inhibits IL-6 function by blocking IL-6 binding to both membrane-bound and soluble forms of IL-6R.[12]

CLINICAL USE OF A HUMANIZED ANTI-INTERLEUKIN-6R ANTIBODY

Katsume and colleagues[13] confirmed the efficacy of a rat anti-mouse IL-6R antibody, MR16-1, in a Castleman disease model mouse, which was a human IL-6 transgenic mouse. After administering MR16-1 into the IL-6 transgenic mouse, most disease symptoms improved without significant side effects. These results underlined the potential for clinical application of anti-IL-6R antibody therapy (**Fig. 4**B).

Permission to treat MCD patients was obtained from the ethics committee of Osaka University. Seven patients with plasma cell variant or the mixed variant MCD were administered with 50 or 100 mg tocilizumab (MRA) once or twice a week. Once

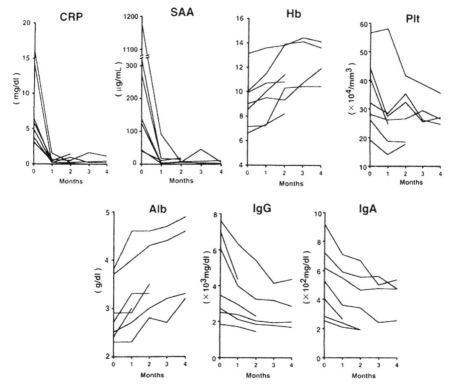

Fig. 6. Courses of laboratory data from 7 MCD patients treated with MRA for 4 months. CRP, SAA, Hb, platelets (Plt), albumin (Alb), immunoglobulin G (IgG), and immunoglobulin A (IgA) are shown. (*Modified from* Nishimoto N, Sasai M, Shima Y, et al. Improvement in Castleman's disease by humanized anti-interleukin-6 receptor antibody therapy. Blood 2000;95(1):59; with permission.)

therapy began, patients' fever ceased, and CRP, fibrinogen, anemia,[14] and albumin started to improve (**Fig. 6**).[15] These therapeutic effects did not diminish after 1 year of continuous treatment. An improvement in lymphadenopathy was also observed in all these patients with a significant reduction in size and in follicular hyperplasia and vascularity (**Fig. 7**B). Skin lesions are one of the characteristic symptoms of MCD. **Fig. 7**C shows a patient with Castleman disease, who had a reddish purple–colored red-skin eruption on the back, which improved in both size and color after therapy with MRA. The pathophysiologic significance of IL-6 in Castleman disease was thus demonstrated. Furthermore, by understanding the pathophysiologic mechanism of MCD, inhibiting IL-6 signaling using MRA was proven to have potential as a new therapy for MCD. A follow-up study is currently ongoing to determine the long-term prognosis of patients treated with MRA.

CLINICAL STUDY OF TOCILIZUMAB OR SILTUXIMAB FOR MULTICENTRIC CASTLEMAN DISEASE THERAPY

This long-term clinical study was designed as a 13-multicenter, open-label trial. Twenty-eight patients were treated with 8 mg/kg MRA every 2 weeks for 16 weeks. Then, patients were enrolled in an open-label extension study.[16] The primary end point was an improvement in disease activity assessed by CRP, SAA, hemoglobin (Hb), and albumin levels. General fatigue was measured using a visual analogue scale (VAS). The results showed that swollen lymph nodes reduced from 13.5 mm to 9.1 mm at 16 weeks and to 8.6 mm at 1 year of short axis (**Fig. 7**A). Mean changes in laboratory tests are shown in **Fig. 8** and **Table 2**. MRA treatments remarkably improved anemia, hypoalbuminemia, and polyclonal hypergammaglobulinemia. Fatigue measured by VAS showed improvements at weeks 6 to 60, and body weight and body mass index

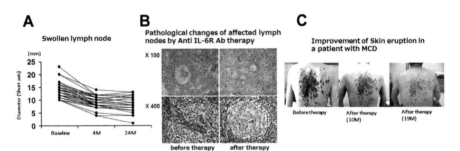

Fig. 7. (*A*) Swollen lymph nodes decrease in size after 4 and 24 months of treatment with MRA; examined using computed tomography. The lymph nodes exceeding 10 mm at baseline were examined from 28 patients. (*B*) The pathologic change of affected lymph node treated with MRA. Enlarged germinal center, numerous plasma cells at interfollicular space and infiltration of vascularity into the germinal center were observed before therapy. After therapy, it diminished the germinal center and follicles in size, and it reduced plasma cells in number. Infiltrated vascularity at the germinal center disappeared; instead, regenerated red deposit was observed after therapy, possibly due to apoptosis. (*C*) Change of skin lesion by MRA therapy. Purple-red skin eruptions on patient's back gradually improved after 10 and 19 months. Color changed from purple-red to light brown with size reduction. ([*A*] *Modified from* Nishimoto N, Kanakura Y, Aozasa K, et al. Humanized anti-interleukin-6 receptor antibody treatment of multicentric Castleman's disease. Blood 2005;106(8):2629, with permission; and [*B*] *Modified from* Nishimoto N, Sasai M, Shima Y, et al. Improvement in Castleman's disease by humanized anti-interleukin-6 receptor antibody therapy. Blood 2000;95(1):59, with permission.)

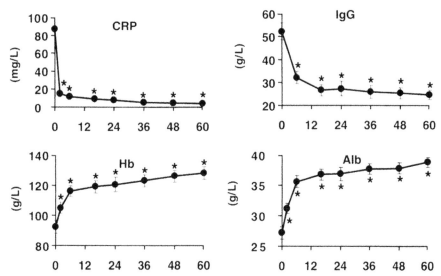

Fig. 8. Courses of laboratory data from 28 MCD patients treated with 8 mg/kg of anti Il-6R antibody every 2 weeks for 60 weeks for 60 weeks, showing CRP, IgG, Hb, and Alb levels. Points and vertical bars indicate mean and standard errors, respectively. IgG gradually decreased; Hb and Alb gradually increased into the normal range. *P < 0.01, paired test compared with baseline. (*Modified from* Nishimoto N, Kanakura Y, Aozasa K, et al. Humanized anti-interleukin-6 receptor antibody treatment of multicentric Castleman's disease. Blood 2005;106(8):2630; with permission.)

Table 2
Mean values for laboratory tests at baseline and at weeks 16 and 60

Measure	Baseline	Week 16	Week 60[a]
Fibrinogen level, mg/dL	639 ± 36	317 ± 28[b]	317 ± 22[b]
ESR, mm/h	114 ± 7	48 ± 8[b]	40 ± 7[b]
HDL cholesterol level, mg/dL	36.1 ± 2.4	52.7 ± 5.3[b]	49.4 ± 3.0[b]
LDL cholesterol level, mg/dL	71.4 ± 4.6	106.5 ± 4.9[b]	109.5 ± 5.9[b]
Triglyceride level, mg/dL	54 ± 4	121 ± 15[b]	138 ± 19[b]
Body weight, kg	56.3 ± 2.0	60.1 ± 2.2	61.0 ± 2.3
BMI	21.6 ± 0.6	23.1 ± 0.6[b]	23.4 ± 0.6[b]
General fatigue, mm (VAS)	29.9 ± 4.3	17.7 ± 3.2[c]	20.4 ± 3.8
IgA, g/L	3.2 ± 0.31	2.47 ± 0.29[b]	2.26 ± 0.21[b]
IgM, g/L	7.1 ± 0.73	3.44 ± 0.38[b]	3.30 ± 0.33[b]
IgE, mg/L	5.0 ± 1.05	4.64 ± 1.62	3.99 ± 0.92[b]

Values are expressed as mean ± standard error. To convert fibrinogen from milligrams per deciliter to micromoles per liter, multiply milligrams per deciliter by 0.0249. To convert HDL and LDL cholesterol from milligrams per deciliter to millimoles per liter, multiply milligrams per deciliter by 0.02586. To convert triglyceride from milligrams per deciliter to millimoles per liter, multiply milligrams per deciliter by 0.0113.

Abbreviations: ESR, erythrocyte sedimentation rate; HDL, high-density lipoprotein; LDL, low-density lipoprotein.

[a] Patients treated with MRA up to 16 weeks (n = 28) and up to 60 weeks (n = 27).
[b] P<.001; paired t test compared with baseline.
[c] P = .008; paired t test compared with baseline.

Modified from Nishimoto N, Kanakura Y, Aozasa K, et al. Humanized anti-interleukin-6 receptor antibody treatment of multicentric Castleman's disease. Blood 2005;106(8):2630; with permission.

Table 3
Body weight and body mass index improvement of underweight patients with Anti IL-6 receptor antibody treatment

Patient	Body Weight, kg			BMI		
	0 wk	16 wk	60 wk	0 wk	16 wk	60 wk
1	43.9	53.3	55.2	16.1	19.6	20.3
2	43.0	55.0	55.0	16.4	21.0	21.0
3	43.6	45.2	48.0	17.5	18.1	19.2
4	51.6	56.3	60.1	18.5	20.1	21.7
5	40.8	41.7	43.8	17.1	17.5	18.4

Five out of 28 patients had BMIs <18.5 and were considered underweight at baseline. Weight gain and improvement were observed with Anti IL-6 receptor antibody treatment in the severe nutritional patients.

Modified from Nishimoto N, Kanakura Y, Aozasa K, et al. Humanized anti-interleukin-6 receptor antibody treatment of multicentric Castleman's disease. Blood 2005;106(8):2631; with permission.

(BMI) gradually improved up to week 60 (**Table 3**). In conclusion, MRA therapy improved the symptoms, laboratory parameters, and lymphadenopathy in MCD patients and the efficacy was maintained or improved over the course of 1 year. The safety profile was acceptable relative to the clinical benefits provided.

In a postmarketing clinical study on the efficacy and safety of 8 mg/kg of tocilizumab in MCD in Japan by Kawabata and colleagues,[17] 11 out of 12 cases achieved partial remission at 2 weeks after treatment, and 3 cases achieved complete remission of all MCD-related symptoms, including lymphadenopathy, hypoalbuminemia, anemia, and a high level of serum CRP. From this sample of 12 MCD patients, 8 were treated with tocilizumab for more than 1 year; their mean Hb levels improved from 7.4 to 12.2 g/dL; serum albumin levels improved from 2.5 to 3.8 g/dL, and serum CRP went from 13.2 to 0.4 mg/dL. Tocilizumab treatment was discontinued because of infection (n = 1) and allergic reaction (n = 1) but was resumed after these symptoms were resolved. Four out of 12 patients completed 6 years of tocilizumab treatment without any adverse events. Although the number of patients was not ideal, this study suggests that tocilizumab is effective and has an acceptable toxicity profile in a real-life clinical setting.

A report that reexamined the application of tocilizumab (MRA, Actemura) was disclosed in 2016 by Pharmaceuticals and Medical Devices Agency (PMDA) in Japan.[18] The report summarized data for 381 MCD patients who were treated with tocilizumab

Table 4
Course of clinical findings after the tocilizumab treatment of multicentric Castleman disease in Japan (mean value of 384 patients)

	2 wk	4 wk–12 wk	15 wk–156 wk
CRP (mg/dL)	<2.0	<2.0	<2.0
Fib (mg/dL)	Decrease	<400	<400
ESR (mm/h)	Gradually decrease		<50
Hb (g/dL)	Gradually increase		<12.0
Alb (g/dL)	Gradually increase		<3.5

Abbreviations: Alb, albumin; ESR, erythrocyte sedimentation rate; Fib, fibrinogen.

From Pharmaceuticals and Medical Devices Agency (PMDA). Tocilizumab re-examination application report for multicentric Castleman disease in Japan. 2017. Available at: http://www.pmda.go.jp/drugs_reexam/2016/P20161005001/450045000_21900AMX01337_A100_1.pdf. Accessed October 6, 2017; with permission.

Table 5
Clinical improvement of symptoms of Castleman disease until 156 weeks in 384 patients treated with tocilizumab

	Improved Case/Objective Case	Improving Rate (%)
Hepatomegaly	35/93	37.6
Splenomegaly	58/145	40.0
Pneumonitis	59/147	40.1
Skin eruption	55/81	67.9
Neurologic disorder	11/22	50.0
Secondary amyloidosis	10/16	62.5
Gastrointestinal Kidney	$\left(\begin{array}{c} 7/11 \\ 3/5 \end{array} \right)$	$\left(\begin{array}{c} 63.6 \\ 60.0 \end{array} \right)$
Lymph node enlargement	53/90	58.9
Undetectable Half size	$\left(\begin{array}{c} 14/90 \\ 39/90 \end{array} \right)$	$\left(\begin{array}{c} 15.6 \\ 43.3 \end{array} \right)$

Hepatomegaly splenomegaly was detected by computed tomography (CT). Pneumonitis was confirmed by CT. Amyloid A amyloidosis was confirmed by the biopsy at pylorus or duodenum, and kidney. Lymph node size was detected by CT.

From Pharmaceuticals and Medical Devices Agency (PMDA). Tocilizumab re-examination application report for multicentric Castleman disease in Japan. 2017; with permission.

at a dose of 8 mg/kg every 2 weeks from 2005 to 2014. Efficacy was analyzed in 354 patients, and the laboratory data for CRP, fibrinogen, Hb, and albumin levels as well as patients' general status were recorded for 156 weeks. A summary of this data can be found in **Table 4**, and patients' physical states and symptoms are shown in **Table 5**. Because of the promising nature of the data, PMDA deemed tocilizumab therapy to be efficacious and safe and approved its use in the treatment of MCD in Japan.

Siltuximab, another IL-6 blocking antibody targeting IL-6 itself, has also demonstrated clinical efficacy leading to resolution of systemic symptoms. A randomized, double-blind, phase 2 trial of siltuximab in at a dose of 11 mg/kg every 3 weeks 79 patients with idiopathic MCD (iMCD) demonstrated significant benefits such as improvements in anemia, inflammatory markers, and systemic symptoms.[19]

SUMMARY

The progress being made in understanding the mechanism of IL-6 and Castleman disease is of interest to researchers and clinicians in the field of hematology, oncology rheumatology, and clinical immunology. In 1982, Yoshizaki and colleagues[1], was the first to identify a T-cell humoral factor that induces B-cell differentiation and assigned it the term "B-cell differentiation factor." In 1986, Hirano and colleagues[3] provided further proof of the molecule, which they referred to as "B-cell stimulatory factor-2" (BSF-2; later changed to IL-6). In 1989, Yoshizaki and colleagues suggested that continuous production of IL-6 was the primary pathogenic event that induced most symptoms and abnormal findings in plasma cell variant Castleman disease. Later, in 2002, after a humanized anti-IL-6 receptor antibody (MRA) was generated by Kishimoto and colleagues and Chugai Pharmaceutical Co., MRA (name later changed to tocilizumab) was first used as a therapeutic agent for the multicentric plasma variant Castleman disease (MCD). Evaluation of pharmacokinetic/pharmacodynamics characteristics, clinical efficacy, and safety has shown that tocilizumab is an important advance in MCD treatment. Tocilizumab monotherapy has demonstrated similar efficacy and safety. Current data suggest that tocilizumab is particularly beneficial in patients who respond inadequately to steroid and other immune suppressants. Hence, tocilizumab might be effective for iMCD patients in whom etiologic cause is still unknown, with significant systemic inflammatory responses and severe anemia or secondary amyloidosis (**Fig. 9**).

Comparative evaluation of the effects of tocilizumab and tumor necrosis factor-α (TNF-α) inhibitors (TNFIs) found that significant improvements in anemia, MCD disease activity (increased level of CRP, and VEGF), and reduction in the serum level of hepcidin were more pronounced in tocilizumab-treated patients than in TNFIs-treated patients in rheumatoid arthritis.[20] Further studies are necessary to fully compare the effect of tocilizumab and TNFIs on MCD anemia and disease activity. In fact, VEGF may play an important role in the vascularity of enlarged lymph nodes in both unicentric and multicentric Castleman disease. Angiogenesis in lymph nodes, which may be regulated by angiogenetic factors, such as VEGF, FGF, PDGF, and some chemokines, is a characteristic pathologic feature of MCD. Blocking the IL-6 pathway with tocilizumab decreases VEGF production, which, in turn, inhibits angiogenesis in lymph node tissues in both unicentric and multicentric Castleman disease. Proteinuria and nephropathy associated with MCD pose other problems. Continuous hyperproduction of SAA (an acute phase protein and a precursor of AA amyloid protein) induced by IL-6 is a cause of kidney disorder due to deposit of AA amyloid protein in the interstitial space of kidney. Suppressing SAA induction by inhibiting IL-6 with tocilizumab delivers rapid results, and the continuous inhibition of IL-6 signaling decreases the deposit of AA amyloid protein in the kidney and gastrointestinal tract.[21] As a result, renal function tends to improve in most MCD patients or elevation of creatinine is halted. These effects have spared some of these MCD patients from having to undergo hemodialysis.

Although IL-6 signaling inhibitors such as tocilizumab and siltuximab have been proven effective for treating MCD, some patients are still resistant to IL-6 inhibition by antibodies. Rapamycin therapy has shown efficacy in treating such severe and resistant patients. In this capacity, rapamycin functions by inhibiting mTORC1, which allows the PI3K-Akt axis activated by IL-6 stimulation to be inhibited by rapamycin. Interestingly, mTORC1 is reported to phosphorylate and activate STAT 3, the major downstream target of IL-6. Therefore, it appears that rapamycin can serve as a therapeutic alternative to IL-6 inhibitors.

Finally, a Jak inhibitor, an intracellular mediator of IL-6, is another therapeutic agent that targets MCD. Actually, tofacitinib, a Jak 1, Jak 2, and Jak 3 inhibitor, is used in rheumatoid arthritis therapy, and its efficacy is comparable to IL-6 or TNF-α inhibitors.

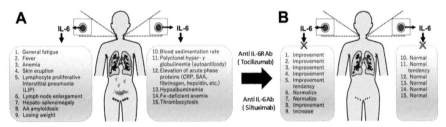

Fig. 9. (*A*) Most abnormal findings could be attributed to the continuous hyperfunction of IL-6 in MCD. IL-6 is produced from affected enlarged lymph node in MCD. IL-6 may induce multiple symptoms and abnormal laboratory findings. (*B*) Most abnormal findings are improved by IL-6 antagonists, such as anti-IL-6R antibody (tocilizumab) or anti-IL-6 antibody (siltuximab) in MCD.

In closing, the progress being made in understanding the mechanism of IL-6 and Castleman disease is of interest to researchers and clinicians in the field of hematology, oncology, rheumatology, and clinical immunology. The more information that can be uncovered through research about IL-6, the causes of IL-6 induction, the pathogenesis of MCD, and the mechanisms that make the current treatment agents (tocilizumab and siltuximab) effective, the more opportunity for improving therapeutic options for MCD patients.

ACKNOWLEDGMENTS

The authors thank Ms Shoko Yamamoto for her secretarial assistance and Ms Leeja Russell for her help in editing the article.

REFERENCES

1. Yoshizaki K, Nakagawa T, Kaieda T, et al. Induction of proliferation and Igs-production in human B leukemic cells by anti-immunoglobulins and T cell factors. J Immunol 1982;128:1296–301.
2. Yoshizaki K, Nakagawa T, Fukunaga K, et al. Isolation and characterization of B cell differentiation factor (BCDF) secreted from a human B lympho-blastoid cell line. J Immunol 1984;132:2948–54.
3. Hirano T, Yasukawa K, Harada H, et al. Complementary DNA for a novel human interleukin (BSF-2) that induces B lymphocytes to produce immunoglobulin. Nature 1986;324:73–6.
4. Hagihara K, Nishikawa T, Sugamata Y, et al. Essential role of STAT3 in cytokine-driven NF-κB-mediated serum amyloid A gene expression. Genes Cells 2005;10:1051–63.
5. Nishikawa T, Hagihara K, Isobe T, et al. Transcriptional Complex formation of c-Fos, STAT3, and hepatocyte NF-1α is essential for cytokine-driven C-reactive protein gene expression. J Immunol 2008;180:3492–501.
6. Song NS, Tomosugi N, Kawabata H, et al. Down-regulation of hepcidin resulting from long-term treatment with an anti-IL-6 receptor antibody (Tocilizumb) improves anemia of inflammation in multicentric Castleman's disease. Blood 2010;116(18):3627–34.
7. Rose-John S. IL-6 trans-signaling via the soluble IL-6 receeptor: importance for the pro-inflammatory activities of IL-6. Int J Biol Sci 2012;8(9):1237–47.
8. Castleman B, Iverson L, Menendez VP. Localized mediastinal lymphnode hyperplasia resembling thymoma. Cancer 1956;9:822.
9. Frizzera G, Peterson BA, Bayrd ED, et al. A systemic lymphoproliferative disorder with morphologic features of Castleman's disease: clinical findings and clinico-pathologic correlations in 15 patients. J Clin Oncol 1985;3:1202.
10. Yoshizaki K, Matsuda T, Nishimoto N, et al. Pathogenic significance of interleukin 6 (IL-6/BSF-2) in Castleman's disease. Blood 1989;74:1360–7.
11. Kishimoto T, Akira S, Taga T. IL-6 receptor and mechanism of signal transduction. Int J Immunopharmacol 1992;14:431–8.
12. Sato K, Tsuchiya M, Saldanh J, et al. Reshaping a human antibody to inhibit the interleukin-6-de-pendent tumor cell growth. Cancer Res 1993;53:851–6.
13. Katsume A, Saito H, Yamada Y, et al. Anti-interleukin 6 (IL-6) receptor antibody suppresses Castleman's disease like symptoms emerged in IL-6 transgenic mice. Cytokine 2002;20:304–11.

14. Song NS, Kazuyuki Y. Up-regulation of hepcidin by interleukin-6 contributes to anemia of inflammation in multicentric Castleman's disease (MCD). Inflamm Regen 2012;32(3):99–106.
15. Nishimoto N, Sasai M, Shima Y, et al. Improvement in Castleman's disease by humanized anti-interleukin-6 receptor antibody therapy. Blood 2000;95:56–61.
16. Nishimoto N, Kanakura Y, Aozasa K, et al. Humanized anti-interleukin-6 receptor antibody treatment of multicentric Castleman's disease. Blood 2005;106: 2627–32.
17. Kawabata H, Kadowaki N, Nishikori M, et al. Clinical features and treatment of multicentric Castleman's disease : a retrospective study of 21 Japanese patients at a single institute. J Clin Exp Hematop 2013;53(1):69–77.
18. Report of clinical study of tocilizumub therapy to multi centric Castleman's disease in Japan. Pharmaceuticals and Medical Devices Agency (PMDA) in Japan. Available at: http://www.pmda.go.jp/drugs_reexam/2016/P20161005001/450045000_21900AMX01337_A100_1.pdf. Accessed August 8, 2017.
19. Van Rhee F, Wong RS, Munshi N, et al. Siltuximub for multi centric Castleman's disease: a randomized, double-blind, placebo- controlled trial. Lancet Oncol 2014;15:966–74.
20. Song NS, Iwahashi M, Tomosugi N, et al. Comparative evaluation of the effects of treatment with tocilizumab and TNF-α inhibitors on serum hepcidin, anemia response and disease activity in rheumatoid arthritis patients. Arthritis Res Ther 2013;15:R141.
21. Yoshizaki K. Basic and clinical significance of interleukin 6 (IL-6) in AA amyloidosis. In: Hazenberg BPC, Bijzet J, editors. XIIIth International Symposium on Amyloidosis. Groningen: Groningen Unit for Amyloidosis Research & Development; 2013. p. 394–7.

Pathology of Castleman Disease

David Wu, MD, PhD[a],*, Megan S. Lim, MD, PhD[b], Elaine S. Jaffe, MD[c]

KEYWORDS

- Pathology • Castleman disease • Hyaline-vascular • Hypervascular
- Plasmacytic features • HHV8/KSHV • TAFRO

KEY POINTS

- The term Castleman disease encompasses several distinct lymphoproliferative disorders, with different underlying disease pathogenesis and clinical outcomes.
- There are three general histologic patterns encountered in Castleman disease: (1) hyaline-vascular occurring in unicentric disease, and (2) hypervascular and (3) plasma cell rich, mainly encountered in patients with multicentric disease; admixed hypervascular and plasmacytic features may be seen.
- HHV8-positive Castleman disease nearly always presents with multicentric disease; HHV8-infected plasmablasts are most often found in the mantle or marginal zones of lymph nodes, and exhibit lambda light chain restriction.
- Thrombocytopenia, ascites/anasarca, myelofibrosis/fever, renal dysfunction/reticulin fibrosis, and organomegaly (TAFRO) represents a distinct clinicopathologic form of idiopathic HHV8/KSHV-negative Castleman disease with mixed hypervascular and plasmacytic histologic features within involved lymph nodes, but additionally has loose bone marrow fibrosis, megakaryocytic hyperplasia, and other syndromic features.

INTRODUCTION

The term Castleman disease has been applied to several different lymphoproliferatiive disorders comprising of several distinct clinicopathologic entities.[1–4] Its prevalence has been estimated recently based on medical insurance claims to be ~21 to 25 cases per million person-years,[5] and thus qualifying it as an orphan disease. The disease presents clinically as unicentric or multicentric in nature[2,3,6,7] (**Table 1**). In the unicentric variant of Castleman, patients have localized disease affecting only a single, enlarged lymph node, or at most a group of adjacent nodes in a single region, with

[a] Department of Laboratory Medicine, University of Washington, 825 Eastlake Avenue East, Room G-7800, Seattle, WA 98109, USA; [b] Department of Pathology and Laboratory Medicine, Perelman School of Medicine University of Pennsylvania, 3400 Civic Center Boulevard, Philadelphia, PA 19104, USA; [c] Laboratory of Pathology, Hematopathology Section, Center for Cancer Research, National Cancer Institute, 10 Center Drive, Room 3S 235, Bethesda, MD 20892, USA
* Corresponding author.
E-mail address: dwu2@uw.edu

Hematol Oncol Clin N Am 32 (2018) 37–52
https://doi.org/10.1016/j.hoc.2017.09.004
0889-8588/18/© 2017 Elsevier Inc. All rights reserved.

Table 1
Clinical variants of Castleman disease and key features

Clinical Variant	Histologic Variant	Key Microscopic Changes	Laboratory Abnormalities	Disease Aggressiveness
Unicentric	Hyaline-vascular (~90%) and plasma cell (10%)	Atretic follicles with hyalinization, and lymphodepletion; concentric "onion-skin" appearance of circumferential mantle zone cells; penetrating vessels imparting "lollipop" appearance; proliferation of vasculature; unapparent sinuses	Limited	Surgical resection is typically curative with excellent outcome
Multicentric	Hypervascular or plasmacytic variant, or commonly mixed	Similar histologic features as hyaline-vascular unicentric Castleman, but typically without dysplastic follicular dendritic cells	Dysregulation of IL-6 (increased) or other cytokines, such as VEGF, IL-1, TNF-α	Can be life-threatening with end-organ damage and failure
		Diffuse proliferation of plasma cells and hyperplastic germinal centers, preserved sinuses		
HHV8-positive Castleman disease	Plasma cell rich	Evidence of HHV8 infection of plasmablasts present in mantle zones with lambda light chain restriction polyclonal plasmacytosis present		Can be aggressive with disease progression to HHV8-positive large B-cell lymphoma
TAFRO	Mixed hypervascular and plasmacytic change	Hypervascular lymph nodal changes and bone marrow reticulin fibrosis with megakaryocytic hyperplasia and emperipolesis	Thrombocytopenia, no hypergammoglobulinemia as frequently seen in idiopathic multicentric Castleman disease	Prolonged course, with occasional flares that can be aggressive and fatal

Abbreviations: HHV8, human herpes virus 8; IL, interleukin; TAFRO, thrombocytopenia, ascites/anasarca, myelofibrosis/reticulin fibrosis, and organomegaly; TNF, tumor necrosis factor; VEGF, vascular endothelial growth factor.

the mediastinum and other thoracic lymph nodes being commonly involved. Patients typically lack significant systemic symptoms and their clinical outcomes are generally favorable with limited morbidity and surgical resection being essentially curative.[8] By contrast, in multicentric Castleman disease, there is diffuse lymphadenopathy affecting multiple groups of lymph nodes in association with marked systemic inflammatory symptoms.[1] The cause of multicentric disease is multifactorial[3] and may in many patients be idiopathic. In patients in whom infection by human herpes virus 8 (HHV8; also known as Kaposi sarcoma herpes virus [KSHV]), is established, a viral cause is clear. However, in cases in which HHV8 infection is absent, the underlying cause is currently unknown with the possible etiologies hypothesized to occur at an intersection of rheumatology, infectious disease, and oncology (**Box 1**).[3] Irrespective of the pathogenesis, multicentric Castleman disease is commonly associated with constitutional symptoms (eg, night sweats, fever, weight loss) and systemic cytokine dysregulation,[9] resulting in prominent abnormal blood count and chemistry, hepatosplenomegaly, and complex organ dysfunction. In some patients, the disease may be particularly aggressive and progress to multiorgan dysfunction and in some individuals, death.[2]

The term Castleman disease has its origins in a case report published in 1954 by the pathologist by Dr. Benjamin Castleman.[10] This initial case report was soon followed by more detailed analysis of patients having isolated mediastinal lymphadenopathy.[10,11] In these initial publications, Castleman and colleagues[11] described what is currently appreciated as unicentric disease with hyaline-vascular histopathologic features. Further work by Keller and coworkers[12] subsequently demonstrated that the

---

Box 1
Potential clinical and histopathologic mimics of Castleman disease

Autoimmune diseases

Rheumatoid arthritis/juvenile idiopathic arthritis

IgG4-related disease

Systemic lupus erythematosus

Hemophagocytic lymphohistiocytosis/macrophage activation syndrome

Adult-onset Still disease

Autoimmune lymphoproliferative syndrome

Infections

Acute Epstein-Barr virus infection

Acute human immunodeficiency virus infection

HHV8/KSHV infection

Other (cytomegalovirus, toxoplasmosis, tuberculosis)

Malignancies

Lymphoma including Hodgkin and non-Hodgkin

Follicular dendritic cell sarcoma

Plasma cell neoplasm, including POEMS

Adapted from Fajgenbaum DC, Uldrick TS, Bagg A, et al. International, evidence-based consensus diagnostic criteria for HHV-8-negative/idiopathic multicentric Castleman disease. Blood 2017;129(12):1652; with permission.

histologic features of unicentric disease could also include plasmacytosis. The uncommon plasma cell form of unicentric Castleman disease was more often associated with systemic symptoms.[12] In subsequent reports published in the late 1970s and early 1980s, the multicentric variant of Castleman was described, demonstrating the propensity of this disease variant to include severe clinical symptomatology with diffuse lymphadenopathy.[12–15] That these patients could be quite sick was a key clinical feature of this multicentric variant of Castleman disease.

In the 1980s, significant insights regarding the pathogenesis of Castleman disease were gained, when Yoshizaki and colleagues[16] identified elevation of the key cytokine interleukin-6 (IL-6) in patients with Castleman disease. This observation along with discoveries by others collectively paved the way for preclinical experimental investigation into the biology and pathogenesis of Castleman disease. With the establishment of IL-6 dysregulation (abnormally increased) in some patients with Castleman disease, the role of this key cytokine in the pathogenesis of some cases of Castleman disease was highlighted. Exogenous expression of IL-6 in murine models led to a lymphoproliferative disorder that mimicked the typical histologic features seen in resected lymph nodes of patients with Castleman disease.[17] In the 1990s, identification of Kaposi sarcoma–associated herpesvirus-like DNA in patients with Castleman disease further led to confirmation of the hypothesis that some aspects of Castleman changes were driven by IL-6, because it was soon appreciated that a viral homologue of IL-6 was produced by KSHV/HHV8-infected cells.[18–21] These insights together led to evaluation of the clinical efficacy of targeting of IL-6 through the use of monoclonal antibodies. Clinical trials were soon performed, resulting in subsequent approval of anti-IL-6 therapies.[22–26] Since then, insight into Castleman disease pathogenesis has steadily increased in time as evidenced by the ever increasing number of publications on this topic.

The term "Castleman disease" has come to be associated with several distinct clinical syndromes and disease entities, which broadly speaking are referred to as unicentric versus multicentric Castleman (**Fig. 1**). The histologic features of unicentric hyaline-vascular disease remain largely unchanged since the original descriptions by Castleman and colleagues in the 1950s, and as a disease entity, is distinct from the more complex clinical syndromes referred to as multicentric Castleman disease. Although historical approaches for subclassifying multicentric

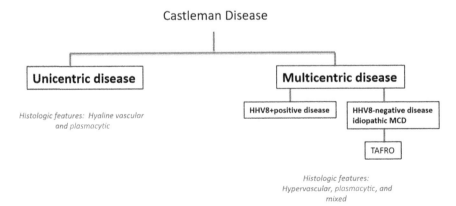

Fig. 1. Clinical variants (*bold*) of Castleman disease and correlated histopathologic patterns (*italicized*). TAFRO, thrombocytopenia, ascites/anasarca, myelofibrosis/fever, renal dysfunction/reticulin fibrosis, and organomegaly. MCD, multicentric castleman disease.

Castleman disease had previously segregated cases based on association with infection by human immunodeficiency virus (HIV), this approach was revised when research showed the critical role of KSHV/HHV8 in this disease, irrespective of HIV infection.[18,27] Accordingly the current diagnostic pathologic paradigm considers multicentric Castleman disease to be subdivided based on whether there is HHV8 infection, either as HHV8-positive Castleman disease versus HHV8-negative, idiopathic Castleman disease[3] (see **Fig. 1**). Although each of these clinicopathologic variants has some distinctive histopathologic features, it should be noted that there is significant pathologic overlap between these different variants in the resected lymph node samples, and that histopathologic findings are not specific when interpreted in isolation.

HISTOPATHOLOGIC FEATURES
Unicentric Castleman Disease

In most cases of unicentric Castleman disease, lymph nodes are significantly enlarged (median diameter of ∼6 cm) and have histopathologic features of hyaline-vascular variant[6,12] (**Fig. 2**). Less commonly, in about one-tenth of unicentric cases, lymph nodes in unicentric disease may have marked plasmacytosis[6] that is more commonly seen in multicentric disease. The lymph nodes involved by the hyaline-vascular histologic variant of Castleman disease exhibit follicular and interfollicular changes with the degree of such changes being variable from case to case. In cases in which follicular changes in the lymph node predominate, the lymphoid follicles are highly abnormal in appearance. The follicles may be increased in density and they may be disorganized, but notably appear atretic in nature, being depleted of lymphoid cells, but with notable retention of follicular dendritic cells (see **Fig. 2**A). The mantle zone lymphocytes surrounding the follicles are concentrically arranged, exhibiting a target-like pattern with a broad zone of small, mature lymphocytes with condensed chromatin and minimal cytoplasm, imparting an onion-skin-like appearance (see **Fig. 2**B). Frequently, there may be radially penetrating sclerotic blood vessels that together with the atretic follicles and concentric mantle zones impart a so-called "lollipop" appearance (see **Fig. 2**C). In some cases, there may be two more adjacent, atretic follicles enveloped by a concentric mantle zone and dendritic meshwork, resulting in a histopathology feature commonly referred to by pathologists as "twinning" (see **Fig. 2**D). Within the interfollicular zones of the excised lymph nodes in hyaline-vascular variant, there often is often a marked proliferation of vasculature, resulting from an increase in density of vasculature with prominent endothelial cells, lining these proliferative vascular walls (see **Fig. 2**E). In unicentric hyaline-vascular variant, lymph node sinuses are typically absent or unapparent, which is a distinction from the hypervascular histopathologic variant seen in multicentric Castleman disease (discussed later) in which nodal sinuses are preserved. Peripherally, the lymph node capsule may be slightly thickened and sclerotic. Other pathologic features of the hyaline-vascular variant of Castleman disease include the presence of intermediate-to-large-sized follicular dendritic cells that may show cytologic atypia.[28,29] Although there has not been consistent evidence in the hyaline-vascular variant of unicentric Castleman to show evidence of clonality of B cells or plasma cells by analysis of immunoglobulin (*IGH*) gene rearrangement,[30,31] some groups using special methods have demonstrated genomic evidence to suggest that hyaline vascular Castleman disease may represent the end result of clonal aberrations occurring in nonlymphoid cells, in particular follicular dendritic cells.[32–34] The stromal/dendritic cell elements in hyaline vascular Castleman disease frequently show dysplastic features. In exceptionally rare cases, follicular dendritic cells may

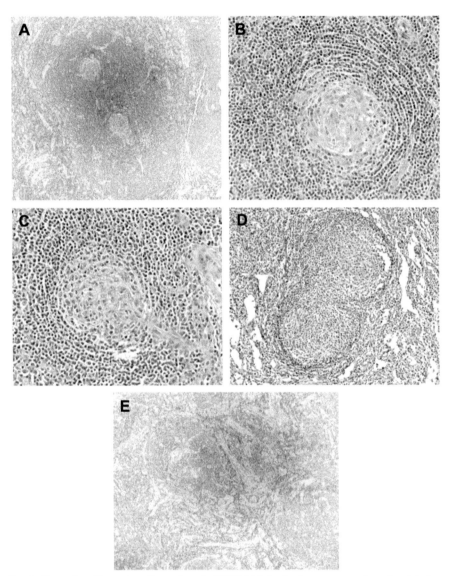

Fig. 2. Example of hematoxylin and eosin (H&E) histologic changes seen in unicentric hyaline vascular and multicentric hypervascular variants. (A) Altered follicles with expanded mantle zones (original magnification ×5). (B) Atretic follicles with mantle zone B cells exhibiting target-like features surrounding residual follicular dendritic cells (original magnification ×20). (C) Radially penetrating sclerotic vasculature (original magnification ×20). (D) Twinning (original magnification ×10). (E) Interfollicular vascular proliferation (original magnification ×5).

be increased in density and proportion, raising concern for a follicular dendritic cell neoplasm. Rarely, such lesions may indeed develop frank morphologic and cytologic atypia of dendritic cells, and be regarded as a follicular dendritic sarcoma.[35,36] Confluent sheets of plasma cells are only rarely seen in unicentric Castleman disease.

By immunohistochemistry, the lymphoid follicles in unicentric hyaline-vascular Castleman disease exhibit significant depletion of follicle centers imparting an atretic appearance. B cells, however, remain present within the expanded mantle zones as evidenced by expression of typical B-cell antigens, such as CD20. These mantle zone cells can further be confirmed by expression of IgD, and using sensitive immunohistochemical techniques may express CD5, an antigen expressed on mantle zone cells in early ontogeny.[37] Although there may be scattered polyclonal plasma cells through the lymph node, large clusters or sheets of plasma cells are not a prominent feature of the hyaline-vascular variant of unicentric Castleman disease. Lastly, atypical dendritic cells within atretic follicles are highlighted by follicular dendritic cell antigens, such as CD21 or CD23.

Rare cases of unicentric Castleman disease ($\sim$10%) exhibit prominent plasmacytosis akin to that seen in multicentric Castleman disease, more typically affecting a group of adjacent lymph nodes rather than a single node.[1,12] Indeed, similar to multicentric Castleman disease, these patients with unicentric disease, but plasma cell-rich histopathology may have significant systemic symptomatology. However, unlike multicentric Castleman, these patients with unicentric disease usually benefit from disease resection with resolution of clinical symptoms.[4,8] Interestingly, such cases may show light chain restriction, with preferential expression of lambda.[37]

Multicentric Castleman Disease

In multicentric Castleman disease, patients typically present with diffuse lymphadenopathy or at a minimum, lymphadenopathy that involves more than one lymph node region. On microscopic examination of excisional lymph node biopsies, there are two common histologic patterns identified: hypervascular and plasmacytic variants. These histologic patterns are not specific or mutually exclusive, because features of either histologic variant may be seen in multicentric Castleman irrespective of cause. These various histologic patterns may also commonly be seen admixed together, and most patients with multicentric Castleman disease show some degree of plasmacytosis.[7]

The hypervascular variant of multicentric Castleman disease[7] is reminiscent in name and histologic features to that of the hyaline-vascular variant of unicentric Castleman disease. A key distinction is that this histopathologic variant is used to describe multicentric Castleman disease in the context of idiopathic multicentric disease with TAFRO syndrome (thrombocytopenia, ascites/anasarca, myelofibrosis/fever, renal dysfunction/reticulin fibrosis, and organomegaly), because of the marked proliferation of the vasculature in this entity. Furthermore, a distinction of the hypervascular variant of multicentric Castleman disease from that of hyaline-vascular variant of unicentric disease is that in the former, lymph node sinuses generally remain patent, whereas lymph node sinuses are absent or not apparent in unicentric Castle disease.[7] The other predominant histologic variant of multicentric Castleman disease is the plasmacytic variant, characterized by the presence of typically large collections or sheets of plasma cells, usually in the absence of regressive changes of follicles and increased vascularity.

Hypervascular variant of multicentric disease

The hypervascular variant of multicentric Castleman disease shares some histopathologic features in common with the unicentric, hyaline-vascular variant of Castleman disease, and was named similarly given the overlap of many histopathologic features commonly observed in the unicentric variant of this disease.[7] The follicles in hypervascular variant of multicentric Castleman disease appear similarly abnormal, principally appearing lymphodepleted with atretic and sclerotic changes being most apparent. Follicle center B cells are diminished in proportion with only residual follicular dendritic cells remaining. Mantle zone B cells may be concentric arranged around the follicles imparting an onion-skin appearance. There is often a marked vascular proliferation in the interfollicular zones with an abundance of high-endothelial venules, and vessels that radially penetrate these atretic follicles, imparting the so-called "lollipop" appearance. One difference between this hypervascular variant and the hyaline-vascular disease of unicentric Castleman disease is the retention of nodal sinuses in multicentric disease versus absence in unicentric disease. In the context of multicentric Castleman disease, particularly the TAFRO variant, some of the distinctive features of hyaline-vascular unicentric disease features, such as the presence of dysplastic follicular dendritic cells, are not observed.[7]

Plasmacytic variant of multicentric disease

This histologic variant is most commonly seen in multicentric Castleman disease and is characterized by the prominence of interfollicular plasma cells within the lymph node (**Fig. 3**). The lymph node architecture is typically preserved with numerous lymphoid follicles showing features of reactive follicular hyperplasia (not shown). The plasma cells are present as large aggregates, or often as confluent sheets, located between the lymphoid follicles (see **Fig. 3**A). The plasma cells are cytologically mature in appearance, without prominent immunoblastic or plasmablastic cytologic features (see **Fig. 3**B). By contrast, plasmablastic cells with prominent nucleoli are not observed unless in the context of KSHV/HHV8 infection, as seen in HHV8-positive Castleman disease. Compared with the hypervascular variant there is less vascular proliferation and hyalination. Although the lymphoid follicles usually appear hyperplastic in nature, typically, in a subset of patients with multicentric disease, there may be some admixed follicles appearing depleted of follicle-center B cells and regressed in nature (see **Fig. 3**A).

By immunohistochemistry, the plasma cells in multicentric Castleman disease are typically polytypic with respect to immunoglobulin light chain expression. By contrast, in HHV8-positive Castleman disease, immunostaining or *in situ*

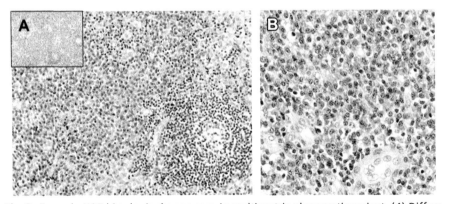

Fig. 3. Example H&E histologic change seen in multicentric plasmacytic variant. (*A*) Diffuse plasmacytosis (original magnification ×10; inset magnification at ×5). (*B*) Mature plasma cells without plasmablasts/immunoblasts. Note the paracoritcal plasmacytosis and in addition, two atretic follicles with slightly expanded mantle zones (original magnification ×40).

hybridization can frequently identify lambda light chain–restricted plasmablasts present within mantle zones with evidence of concurrent infection by HHV8/KSHV.

In patients with idiopathic multicentric Castleman disease the lymph nodes may show variation in the histologic features, so that in any given lymph node biopsy, there may be plasmacytic histology, whereas in other biopsies there may be hypervascular histology.[6,38] Indeed, in some cases of multicentric Castleman disease, there may be histologic features of both the hypervascular variant and the plasmacytic variant, so-called "mixed variant." The significance of the proportion of these different histologic patterns within a given biopsy from a patient with Castleman disease is not clear. Some studies have noted that patients with plasmacytic histology, as compared with the hypervascular histology, have an overall more clinically aggressive course[4] and are less responsiveness to anti-IL-6 therapy.[23] However, these different histologic patterns may be variably seen in the same patient at different times.[7,23] It is likely that these different patterns reflect differences in pathogenesis, because for most cases of idiopathic multicentric Castleman disease, the pathogenesis is unknown.

Thrombocytopenia, ascites/anasarca, myelofibrosis/fever, renal dysfunction/reticulin fibrosis, and organomegaly syndrome

The syndrome of TAFRO is a recently described variant of idiopathic HHV8-negative multicentric Castleman disease,[39–42] occurring in adults (median age ~ 50 years). Although first described in Japan, this variant has since been described in patients of other ethnicities, including white persons.[42] In this variant, there are similar clinicopatho-pathologic features to that of idiopathic multicentric Castleman disease, including involvement of multiple lymph nodes with typical mixed (plasmacytic and hypervascular) histologic features[39] and systemic disease symptomatology. The lymph nodes typically show marked vascular proliferation in the interfollicular areas, and exhibit more a more modest increase in plasma cells. Most follicles often appear atretic and regressed and depleted of germinal center B cells with only remnant dendritic cells. In contrast to that observed in unicentric hyaline-vascular variant, dysplasia of follicular dendritic cells is not seen. Immunostaining for viral markers for HHV8 infection is definitionally negative. Bone marrow core biopsies of patients with TAFRO typically performed to evaluate thrombocytopenia show megakaryocytic hyperplasia with clustering in a background diffuse reticulin fibrosis.[40,42,43] A novel feature is emperipolesis exhibited by megakaryocytes, not encountered in other forms of Castleman disease.

Human Herpes Virus 8-Positive, Castleman Disease

In some patients, many of whom may be immunosuppressed because of HIV infection, HHV-8/KSHV-positive infection can result in a systemic cytokine dysregulation that results in a clinicopathologic picture of multicentric Castleman disease. Although historical classification of multicentric Castleman had initially considered the importance of HIV infection, recognition of the critical role of the HHV-8 virus in these and other patients without HIV infection[18] led to reconsideration of Castleman disease classification on the basis of HHV-8 infection, and not HIV.[3] The histopathologic features of excised lymph nodes are similar to that seen in idiopathic, HHV8-negative multicentric disease with the presence of atretic lymphoid follicles with prominent interfollicular polytypic plasmacytosis.[44] Overall the lymph node architecture is generally preserved. There may be concurrent follicle hyalinization and lymphodepletion with prominent interfollicular vasculature. HHV8-positive/KSHV infected plasmablasts, which are medium-to-large-sized mononuclear cells with amphophilic cytoplasm, may be readily identified within the mantle cell zones surrounding these nodal follicles (**Fig. 4**). In some cases, these plasmablasts may coalesce together,

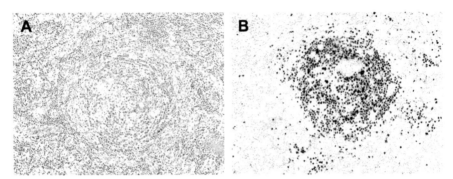

Fig. 4. Example of infection by HHV8 in HHV8-positive multicentric Castleman disease. (*A*) Prominent increase in plasmablasts (H&E, original magnification ×10). (*B*) Immunostaining for HHV8 (latent nuclear antigen-1) (original magnification ×10).

forming prominent aggregates. Immunohistochemical studies show evidence of infection by HHV8/KHSV based on expression of viral proteins, including latent nuclear antigen-1 (see **Fig. 4**B). These cells express B cell and plasma cell markers, including CD20, CD79a, and IRF4/MUM1, but typically lack expression of CD10, PAX5, and BCL6.[44] The plasmablastic cells are typically polyclonal with respect to analysis of immunoglobulin gene rearrangement, but may show IgM lambda light chain restriction. The cause of the preferential expression of lambda light chain in these plasmablastic cells is under current investigation. Some recent studies, summarized by Wang and colleagues,[45] suggest that HHV8 viral transcriptional programming may result in preferential enrichment and/or selection of lambda-expressing plasma cells. In some cases, plasmablasts may aggregate in a manner histologically concerning for malignancy on microscopic examination because of the increased clustering and density. However, the main differential diagnosis in this context is HHV8-positive diffuse large B-cell lymphoma. In contrast, in multicentric Castleman disease, plasmablastic cells are not present in a diffuse sheet-like pattern.[44] In the 2008 World Health Organization classification approach, aggregates of plasmablasts were previously termed so-called "microlymphomas." However, this designation has since been updated in the 2016 World Health Organization revision because of the recognition that not all plasmablastic aggregates are definitively clonal in nature, and that not all plasmablastic proliferations uniformly transform or progress into lymphoma. Nevertheless, in a minor subset of cases, these plasmablasts may acquire additional genomic aberrations, expand in proportion to further more extensively involve the lymph node, and progress to histologically recognizable lymphoma, currently termed HHV8-positive diffuse large B-cell lymphoma.[44]

HISTOLOGIC DIFFERENTIAL DIAGNOSES

Castleman-like histopathologic change may occur in a variety of reactive and neoplastic contexts (see **Box 1**). Accordingly, careful clinicopathologic and laboratory correlation is always required to make a formal diagnosis of Castleman disease. This is true for all histopathologic forms, including the unicentric hyaline-vascular variant, but is typically more critical for the patient with possible multicentric Castleman disease. Hyaline-vascular-like and plasmacytic-like Castleman changes may also be observed in the context of reactive settings (eg, autoimmune disorders, infection), and in some non-Hodgkin lymphomas[46,47] and Hodgkin lymphomas.[48–52] In cases in which there may be concern for lymphoma versus Castleman disease, typically the Castleman-like features are usually limited in nature, not fully involving the lymph node as would happen in true Castleman disease. Importantly, the patient lacks the typical clinical and laboratory picture of Castleman disease. Evidence for the presence of a clonal or light chain–restricted B-cell population by either concurrent molecular analyses of immunoglobulin gene rearrangement or flow cytometry, respectively, provides additional support for the presence of a non-Hodgkin lymphoma. Careful interpretation of histologic features and immunohistochemistry studies is nevertheless required to distinguish nodal involvement by non-Hodgkin or Hodgkin lymphomas from Castleman disease.[53,54] Indeed, according to the recent consensus diagnostic approach, all potential reactive and malignant mimics of Castleman must be excluded before making a diagnosis of idiopathic multicentric Castleman disease.[7] Any diagnosis of Castleman disease should be made using a full excisional lymph node biopsy, because use of only needle-core biopsies is wholly inadequate.

CONSENSUS DIAGNOSTIC CRITERIA FOR HUMAN HERPES VIRUS 8-NEGATIVE, IDIOPATHIC MULTICENTRIC CASTLEMAN DISEASE

In 2015 to 2016, a group of pathologists and clinicians, led by Drs David Fajgenbaum of University of Pennsylvania and Frits van Rhee of University of Arkansas, converged to formulate a systematic review of the criteria for the diagnosis of Castleman disease resulting in the first international consensus diagnostic criteria for idiopathic (HHV8/KSHV-negative) multicentric Castleman disease based on review of 288 clinical cases and 88 tissue samples.[7] This group met to define the diagnostic histopathologic and clinical features of Castleman disease first through informal meetings held concurrently with the annual American Society of Hematology meetings, and second through multiple organized teleconferences and subsequently in-person meetings. During this process, a group of hematopathologists concurrently reviewed numerous Castleman disease cases together with a multiheaded microscope. These cases were derived principally from the cohort of patients with idiopathic HHV8-negative Castleman disease enrolled in the study that resulted in the approval of an anti-IL6 drug,[23] but included numerous, additional cases derived from personal consultative files of participating expert hematopathologists.

Through iterative meetings conducted in person and subsequently virtually, diagnostic histologic and clinical criteria were formulated and agreed on with subsequent submission for external review.[7] The culmination of this extraordinary effort was the development of the first international consensus diagnostic criteria focused on the diagnostic clinicopathologic features of idiopathic (HHV8-negative) multicentric Castleman diseases nearly 70 years after Castleman's original report.[7]

To make a diagnosis of idiopathic multicentric Castleman disease, identification of major and minor clinical and histopathologic criteria is required with exclusion of all reactive, and/or secondary mimics including autoimmune disease and infection.[7] The major criteria require characteristic lymph node histopathology, and evidence of multicentric lymphadenopathy (greater than 1 cm in more than two nodal groups). (**Table 2**). Additionally, 2 of 11 minor criteria must be identified from either laboratory or clinical criteria, with at least one representing a clinical laboratory abnormality. Lastly, exclusion of confounders that may mimic multicentric Castleman disease (see **Box 1**) must be performed. The development of a consensus diagnostic clinicopathologic approach will lead to standardized diagnoses and improvements in understanding of the clinical behavior and response to therapies and disease treatment algorithms.

Table 2
Pathologic diagnostic criteria for HHV8/KSHV-negative idiopathic multicentric Castleman disease

Histologic Features	Spectrum of Changes	Diagnostic Criteria Required
Regressed germinal centers	None > few > many > most	Few or many regressed germinal centers to satisfy major criterion 1 (grade 2–3)
Prominent follicular dendritic cells	None > mild > moderate > very prominent	
Vascularity	Normal > mildly increased > moderately increased > very prominent	
Hyperplastic germinal centers	None > few > many > most	
Plasmacytosis	Normal > mildly > moderately > very increased (sheet-like)	Mildly or moderately increased plasmacytosis to satisfy major criterion 1 (grade 2–3)

For a diagnosis of idiopathic HHV8-negative Castleman disease, cases must satisfy both major criteria and must have at least 2 of 11 potential minor criteria (including at least one laboratory criterion). Major criterion 1 are histopathologic in nature and are detailed above. Major criterion 2 is the presence of enlarged lymph nodes ($\geq$1 cm short axis diameter) in $\geq$2 lymph node stations. Minor criteria include laboratory alterations (elevated C-reactive protein, anemia, thrombocytopenia, hypoalbuminemia, renal dysfunction, polyclonal hypergammaglobulinemia) and clinical findings (constitutional symptoms, hepatosplenomegaly, fluid accumulation, eruptive cherry hemangiomatosis or violaceous papules, lymphocytic interstitial pneumonitis). See Fajgenbaum and coworkers[7] for further details.

Adapted from Fajgenbaum DC, Uldrick TS, Bagg A, et al. International, evidence-based consensus diagnostic criteria for HHV-8-negative/idiopathic multicentric Castleman disease. Blood 2017;129(12):1652; with permission.

SUMMARY AND DISCUSSION

The term Castleman disease has been used to encompass a spectrum of diverse lymphoproliferative disorders with immune perturbations and variable clinical features; disease pathogenesis (although many cases are frequently idiopathic); and as described herein, histopathologic features. The clinicopathologic syndromes may have overlapping histopathologic features, but even these are generally not specific in nature. The most histologically distinctive changes are seen in unicentric Castleman disease of the hyaline-vascular variant. The disease is limited in scope without significant systemic dysfunction or patient morbidity. In multicentric Castleman disease, patients typically exhibit diffuse lymphadenopathy and significant constitutional symptoms, laboratory abnormalities, and hepatosplenomegaly that may result in significant morbidity and mortality. The histologic findings in idiopathic multicentric Castleman disease include hypervascularity (particularly in TAFRO) or marked plasmacytosis, with these two features together bookending the spectrum of histologic changes that may be seen. Frequent admixture of these two histologic patterns along a continuum is observed. The hypervascular variant of multicentric Castleman shares some features with the hyaline-vascular variant of unicentric Castleman, but is distinguished principally by the clinical context (multicentric vs unicentric disease), the presence of patent sinuses in the former and absence in the latter, and absence of dysplastic dendritic cells in hypervascular variant. Additionally, perhaps paradoxically, hyaline vascular Castleman disease usually presents with markedly enlarged lymph nodes resulting in localized mass lesions, whereas the lymph nodes in TAFRO are only moderately enlarged. Additionally, TAFRO presents with thrombocytopenia and loose marrow fibrosis along with nodal Castleman-like changes, in particular hypervascularity. Lymph node changes in TAFRO are characterized by markedly increased vascularity, which extends to the residual follicles, and modest plasmacytosis. In HHV8/KSHV-positive Castleman disease, in addition to marked plasmacytosis, resembling the plasma cell variant, there is notable evidence of HHV8-positive infected plasmablasts within nodal mantle/marginal zones. Lastly, it is important to emphasize that Castleman-like histopathologic changes may be observed in reactive (infectious and autoimmune) disorders, and in malignant lymphomas (non-Hodgkin and Hodgkin lymphoma). Accordingly, careful clinicopathologic correlation is always required to ensure correct diagnoses are made. In this regard, the recent development and publication of international consensus criteria for diagnosing idiopathic, HHV8-negative multicentric variant of Castleman disease should be most helpful.[7]

The increased interest and research into delineating the diagnostic clinicopathologic features of Castleman disease will enable further insight into the disease pathogenesis of the clinicopathologic variants currently grouped together under the eponym of Castleman disease. With further insight into pathogenesis, improved clinical diagnoses may be possible with an expectation that better disease classification and prognostication should contribute to improved patient care.

REFERENCES

1. Frizzera G. Castleman's disease and related disorders. Semin Diagn Pathol 1988; 5(4):346–64.
2. Talat N, Schulte KM. Castleman's disease: systematic analysis of 416 patients from the literature. Oncologist 2011;16(9):1316–24.
3. Fajgenbaum DC, van Rhee F, Nabel CS. HHV-8-negative, idiopathic multicentric Castleman disease: novel insights into biology, pathogenesis, and therapy. Blood 2014;123(19):2924–33.
4. Yu L, Tu M, Cortes J, et al. Clinical and pathological characteristics of HIV- and HHV-8-negative Castleman disease. Blood 2017;129(12):1658–68.
5. Munshi N, Mehra M, van de Velde H, et al. Use of a claims database to characterize and estimate the incidence rate for Castleman disease. Leuk Lymphoma 2015;56(5):1252–60.
6. Cronin DM, Warnke RA. Castleman disease: an update on classification and the spectrum of associated lesions. Adv Anat Pathol 2009;16(4):236–46.
7. Fajgenbaum DC, Uldrick TS, Bagg A, et al. International, evidence-based consensus diagnostic criteria for HHV-8-negative/idiopathic multicentric Castleman disease. Blood 2017;129(12):1646–57.
8. Talat N, Belgaumkar AP, Schulte KM. Surgery in Castleman's disease: a systematic review of 404 published cases. Ann Surg 2012;255(4):677–84.
9. Casper C, Chaturvedi S, Munshi N, et al. Analysis of inflammatory and anemia-related biomarkers in a randomized, double-blind, placebo-controlled study of siltuximab (anti-IL6 monoclonal antibody) in patients with multicentric Castleman disease. Clin Cancer Res 2015;21(19):4294–304.
10. Castleman B, Towne VW. Case records of the Massachusetts General Hospital; weekly clinicopathological exercises; founded by Richard C. Cabot. N Engl J Med 1954;251(10):396–400.

11. Castleman B, Iverson L, Menendez VP. Localized mediastinal lymph node hyperplasia resembling thymoma. Cancer 1956;9(4):822–30.
12. Keller AR, Hochholzer L, Castleman B. Hyaline-vascular and plasma-cell types of giant lymph node hyperplasia of the mediastinum and other locations. Cancer 1972;29(3):670–83.
13. Frizzera G, Banks PM, Massarelli G, et al. A systemic lymphoproliferative disorder with morphologic features of Castleman's disease. Pathological findings in 15 patients. Am J Surg Pathol 1983;7(3):211–31.
14. Frizzera G, Peterson BA, Bayrd ED, et al. A systemic lymphoproliferative disorder with morphologic features of Castleman's disease: clinical findings and clinicopathologic correlations in 15 patients. J Clin Oncol 1985;3(9):1202–16.
15. Gaba AR, Stein RS, Sweet DL, et al. Multicentric giant lymph node hyperplasia. Am J Clin Pathol 1978;69(1):86–90.
16. Yoshizaki K, Matsuda T, Nishimoto N, et al. Pathogenic significance of interleukin-6 (IL-6/BSF-2) in Castleman's disease. Blood 1989;74(4):1360–7.
17. Brandt SJ, Bodine DM, Dunbar CE, et al. Dysregulated interleukin 6 expression produces a syndrome resembling Castleman's disease in mice. J Clin Invest 1990;86(2):592–9.
18. Soulier J, Grollet L, Oksenhendler E, et al. Kaposi's sarcoma-associated herpesvirus-like DNA sequences in multicentric Castleman's disease. Blood 1995;86(4):1276–80.
19. Yabuhara A, Yanagisawa M, Murata T, et al. Giant lymph node hyperplasia (Castleman's disease) with spontaneous production of high levels of B-cell differentiation factor activity. Cancer 1989;63(2):260–5.
20. Leger-Ravet MB, Peuchmaur M, Devergne O, et al. Interleukin-6 gene expression in Castleman's disease. Blood 1991;78(11):2923–30.
21. Aoki Y, Tosato G, Fonville TW, et al. Serum viral interleukin-6 in AIDS-related multicentric Castleman disease. Blood 2001;97(8):2526–7.
22. Beck JT, Hsu SM, Wijdenes J, et al. Brief report: alleviation of systemic manifestations of Castleman's disease by monoclonal anti-interleukin-6 antibody. N Engl J Med 1994;330(9):602–5.
23. van Rhee F, Wong RS, Munshi N, et al. Siltuximab for multicentric Castleman's disease: a randomised, double-blind, placebo-controlled trial. Lancet Oncol 2014;15(9):966–74.
24. Kurzrock R, Voorhees PM, Casper C, et al. A phase I, open-label study of siltuximab, an anti-IL-6 monoclonal antibody, in patients with B-cell non-Hodgkin lymphoma, multiple myeloma, or Castleman disease. Clin Cancer Res 2013;19(13):3659–70.
25. Nishimoto N, Kanakura Y, Aozasa K, et al. Humanized anti-interleukin-6 receptor antibody treatment of multicentric Castleman disease. Blood 2005;106(8):2627–32.
26. Nishimoto N, Terao K, Mima T, et al. Mechanisms and pathologic significances in increase in serum interleukin-6 (IL-6) and soluble IL-6 receptor after administration of an anti-IL-6 receptor antibody, tocilizumab, in patients with rheumatoid arthritis and Castleman disease. Blood 2008;112(10):3959–64.
27. Dossier A, Meignin V, Fieschi C, et al. Human herpesvirus 8-related Castleman disease in the absence of HIV infection. Clin Infect Dis 2013;56(6):833–42.
28. Nguyen DT, Diamond LW, Hansmann ML, et al. Castleman's disease. Differences in follicular dendritic network in the hyaline vascular and plasma cell variants. Histopathology 1994;24(5):437–43.

29. Lin O, Frizzera G. Angiomyoid and follicular dendritic cell proliferative lesions in Castleman's disease of hyaline-vascular type: a study of 10 cases. Am J Surg Pathol 1997;21(11):1295–306.
30. Menke DM, DeWald GW. Lack of cytogenetic abnormalities in Castleman's disease. South Med J 2001;94(5):472–4.
31. Hanson CA, Frizzera G, Patton DF, et al. Clonal rearrangement for immunoglobulin and T-cell receptor genes in systemic Castleman's disease. Association with Epstein-Barr virus. Am J Pathol 1988;131(1):84–91.
32. Chang KC, Wang YC, Hung LY, et al. Monoclonality and cytogenetic abnormalities in hyaline vascular Castleman disease. Mod Pathol 2014;27(6):823–31.
33. Cokelaere K, Debiec-Rychter M, De Wolf-Peeters C, et al. Hyaline vascular Castleman's disease with HMGIC rearrangement in follicular dendritic cells: molecular evidence of mesenchymal tumorigenesis. Am J Surg Pathol 2002;26(5):662–9.
34. Pauwels P, Dal Cin P, Vlasveld LT, et al. A chromosomal abnormality in hyaline vascular Castleman's disease: evidence for clonal proliferation of dysplastic stromal cells. Am J Surg Pathol 2000;24(6):882–8.
35. Chan JK, Tsang WY, Ng CS. Follicular dendritic cell tumor and vascular neoplasm complicating hyaline-vascular Castleman's disease. Am J Surg Pathol 1994; 18(5):517–25.
36. Chan JK, Fletcher CD, Nayler SJ, et al. Follicular dendritic cell sarcoma. Clinicopathologic analysis of 17 cases suggesting a malignant potential higher than currently recognized. Cancer 1997;79(2):294–313.
37. Radaszkiewicz T, Hansmann ML, Lennert K. Monoclonality and polyclonality of plasma cells in Castleman's disease of the plasma cell variant. Histopathology 1989;14(1):11–24.
38. Liu AY, Nabel CS, Finkelman BS, et al. Idiopathic multicentric Castleman's disease: a systematic literature review. Lancet Haematol 2016;3(4):e163–75.
39. Kawabata H, Takai K, Kojima M, et al. Castleman-Kojima disease (TAFRO syndrome): a novel systemic inflammatory disease characterized by a constellation of symptoms, namely, thrombocytopenia, ascites (anasarca), microcytic anemia, myelofibrosis, renal dysfunction, and organomegaly: a status report and summary of Fukushima (6 June, 2012) and Nagoya meetings (22 September, 2012). J Clin Exp Hematop 2013;53(1):57–61.
40. Iwaki N, Sato Y, Takata K, et al. Atypical hyaline vascular-type castleman's disease with thrombocytopenia, anasarca, fever, and systemic lymphadenopathy. J Clin Exp Hematop 2013;53(1):87–93.
41. Masaki Y, Nakajima A, Iwao H, et al. Japanese variant of multicentric castleman's disease associated with serositis and thrombocytopenia: a report of two cases: is TAFRO syndrome (Castleman-Kojima disease) a distinct clinicopathological entity? J Clin Exp Hematop 2013;53(1):79–85.
42. Iwaki N, Fajgenbaum DC, Nabel CS, et al. Clinicopathologic analysis of TAFRO syndrome demonstrates a distinct subtype of HHV-8-negative multicentric Castleman disease. Am J Hematol 2016;91(2):220–6.
43. Hawkins JM, Pillai V. TAFRO syndrome or Castleman-Kojima syndrome: a variant of multicentric Castleman disease. Blood 2015;126(18):2163.
44. Chadburn A, Said J, Gratzinger D, et al. HHV8/KSHV-positive lymphoproliferative disorders and the spectrum of plasmablastic and plasma cell neoplasms: 2015 SH/EAHP workshop report-part 3. Am J Clin Pathol 2017;147(2):171–87.
45. Wang HW, Pittaluga S, Jaffe ES. Multicentric Castleman disease: where are we now? Semin Diagn Pathol 2016;33(5):294–306.

46. Pina-Oviedo S, Wang W, Vicknair E, et al. Follicular lymphoma with hyaline-vascular Castleman disease-like follicles and CD20 positive follicular dendritic cells. Pathology 2017;49(5):544–7.
47. Siddiqi IN, Brynes RK, Wang E. B-cell lymphoma with hyaline vascular Castleman disease-like features: a clinicopathologic study. Am J Clin Pathol 2011;135(6):901–14.
48. Zarate-Osorno A, Medeiros LJ, Danon AD, et al. Hodgkin's disease with coexistent Castleman-like histologic features. A report of three cases. Arch Pathol Lab Med 1994;118(3):270–4.
49. Filliatre-Clement L, Busby-Venner H, Moulin C, et al. Hodgkin Lymphoma and Castleman disease: when one blood disease can hide another. Case Rep Hematol 2017;2017:9423205.
50. Gong S, Hijiya N. Classical Hodgkin lymphoma and Castleman disease: a rare morphologic combination. Blood 2017;130(3):381.
51. Naik LP, Fernandes G, Mahapatra L. Cytology of Castleman disease hyaline vascular type: a close differential diagnosis with Hodgkin's lymphoma. Acta Cytol 2010;54(5 Suppl):1093–4.
52. Maheswaran PR, Ramsay AD, Norton AJ, et al. Hodgkin's disease presenting with the histological features of Castleman's disease. Histopathology 1991;18(3):249–53.
53. Zanetto U, Pagani FP, Perez C. Interfollicular Hodgkin's lymphoma and Castleman's disease. Histopathology 2006;48(3):317–9.
54. Liu Q, Pittaluga S, Davies-Hill T, et al. Increased CD5-positive polyclonal B cells in Castleman disease: a diagnostic pitfall. Histopathology 2013;63(6):877–80.

Diagnosis of Castleman Disease

Raphaël Szalat, MD[a], Nikhil C. Munshi, MD[a,b],*

KEYWORDS

- Castleman disease • Diagnosis • HHV8 • POEMS • TAFRO
- Paraneoplastic pemphigus

KEY POINTS

- Castleman disease (CD) comprises a heterogeneous group of disorders that share pathology similarities but present with diverse clinical manifestations.
- Specific clinical signs and complications, including paraneoplastic pemphigus, peripheral neuropathy, TAFRO (thrombocytopenia, anasarca, fever, reticulin fibrosis, organomegaly) and POEMS (polyradiculoneuropathy, organomegaly, endocrinopathy, monoclonal plasma cell disorder, skin changes) syndrome, or human herpesvirus 8 (HHV8) infection, are important features of CD's clinical spectrum that should be recognized and identified.
- Evaluation of CD should include, besides pathologic evaluation with immunostaining, laboratory investigations as well as systemic imaging with PET/computed tomography, both to stage the extent of disease (unicentric vs multicentric) as well as for markers for follow-up.
- HHV8-related CD requires evaluation for the presence of Kaposi sarcoma and HIV infection and is associated with increased risk of lymphoma.
- Lymphoma and autoimmune connective disorders can present with Castleman-like lymph nodes pathology and need to be excluded.

The original description of Castleman disease (CD), corresponding to the presence of angiofollicular lymph-node hyperplasia with capillary proliferation, hyperplasia of lymphoid follicles, and cellular infiltration of plasma cells, was first reported in 1956 in a series of patients with few or no symptoms but solitary mediastinal lymph node enlargement.[1] Sixty years later, CD remains a rare condition that comprises 3 distinct entities that share pathologic similarities regarding germinal centers, follicular

The authors declare no disclosure of any relationship with a commercial company that has a direct financial interest in subject matter or materials discussed in this article or with a company making a competing product.

[a] Medical Oncology, Dana-Farber Cancer Institute, 450 Brookline Avenue, M230 Boston, MA 02215, USA; [b] VA Boston Healthcare System, 1400 VFW Parkway, West Roxbury, MA, USA
* Corresponding author. Dana Farber Cancer Institute, 450 Brookline Avenue, M230 Boston, MA 02215, USA
E-mail address: Nikhil_Munshi@dfci.harvard.edu

dendritic and plasma cell prominence, and vascularity within lymph nodes but are featured by specific clinical, pathologic, and biological abnormalities. The lack of specificity of most of the pathology and clinical findings observed in CD requires adequate criteria to diagnose CD and rule out differential diagnoses. Multicentric Castleman disease (MCD) is classically distinguished from unicentric Castleman disease (UCD) by the presence of systemic symptoms (fever, asthenia, pleural effusion, ascites), presence of lymph nodes in more than one region, hepatosplenomegaly, and important signs of biological inflammation, as well as a poorer prognosis. MCD comprises 2 subgroups: human herpesvirus 8 (HHV8) -related MCD[2,3] and idiopathic multicentric Castleman disease (iMCD) which is not associated with any known etiologic factor.[4] Here, the authors review the clinical and pathologic situations that should lead to diagnosis of CD.

To establish the diagnosis of CD and specify its subtype, a complete clinical evaluation associated with lymph node biopsy and biological and morphologic examination is necessary. Here, we review the clinical and pathologic situations that should lead to diagnosis of CD.

PRESENTATION

The presentation of CD is varied. In patients with UCD, presentation is quite often asymptomatic with accidental detection of visible or palpable mass (enlarged lymph node) or abnormal laboratory tests on routine or unrelated examination. Rarely, UCD may present with systemic symptoms or because enlarged lymph node may impede nearby organs. On the other hand, MCD often presents with fever, night sweats, weakness, severe fatigue, and anorexia accompanied by weight loss. These classic systemic symptoms of MCD, are considered mainly driven by interleukin-6 (IL-6). Patients may have symptoms associated with complications of CD, including cutaneous, neurologic, or autoimmune manifestations. Because no symptom or laboratory investigation is diagnostic of CD, the ultimate and often the first investigation is lymph node biopsy with careful histologic examination by an experienced pathologist.

HISTOPATHOLOGICAL EXAMINATION OF CASTLEMAN DISEASE

Three distinct subtypes of CD can be distinguished based on lymph node pathology examination (see **Table 1**). Benjamin Castleman's initial report corresponds to the hyalin-vascular subtype, which is the most common feature of UCD.[1,5]

In the hyalin-vascular subtype, the lymph node architecture is featured by lymphoid follicles with atrophic or "regressed" germinal centers often hyalinized and mainly constituted by residual follicular dendritic cells, and prominent mantle zones containing small lymphocytes are seen. The follicular dendritic cells are organized in concentric form and provide an "onion-skin" appearance. Sclerotic blood vessels are often

Table 1 Histologic and clinical subtypes of Castleman disease			
Histologic Lesion	UCD	HHV8-Related MCD	iMCD
Hyaline vascular	++++	+/−	+
Plasmacytic	+	+++	++
Mixed	+/−	++	++

UCD is more often associated with the hyaline-vascular subtype, whereas MCD is more often associated with plasma cell and mixed subtypes. The presence of plasmablast is exclusively observed in the context of HHV8-related MCD.

seen penetrating the atrophic germinal centers, producing so-called lollipop lesions. The interfollicular lymphoid tissue contains numerous small blood vessels. Adjacent germinal centers can be encircled by a single mantle zone, a phenomenon referred to as germinal center "twinning."

In the plasmacytic subtype, the interfollicular regions are hypervascular and infiltrated by numerous plasma cells in sheets, and the lymphoid follicles are inconstantly featured by germinal centers that are either hyperplastic or sometimes coexist with regression. The plasma cell variants are the most common subtype of MCD (75%), but represent 10% to 20% of UCD.[6]

The coexistence of typical hyalin-vascular and plasma cell type refers to a mixed form of CD that is observed in a small subset of UCD but is common in HHV8-related MCD. In this subgroup, in addition to the typical histology of the mixed form, the presence of numerous immunoblasts (also called plasmablasts), which correspond to HHV8-infected B cells (latent nuclear antigen-1 positive staining), is observed in the mantle zone and 40% contain coexistent Kaposi sarcoma.[7] In all subtypes, B cells and plasma cells are polyclonal, but often monotypic, and T cells show no aberrant immunophenotype.

LABORATORY AND RADIOLOGICAL INVESTIGATIONS

The recommended laboratory investigations are directed at detecting and diagnosing the variant of CD (UCD or MCD) and then investigating various clinical and biological effects of CD. The list of the tests and expected abnormalities is presented in **Table 2**. Once biopsy suggests CD, one of the first investigations is radiological survey of lymph nodes to determine whether the patient has UCD or MCD. Either fluorodeoxyglucose-PET/computed tomography (CT) or CT of the neck/chest/abdomen and pelvis can be considered. PET/CT is preferred because it will also identify the relative metabolic activity of the lymph node. In CD, usually the standardized uptake value (SUV) is lower compared with lymphoma, an important distinction to make. Imaging may also help detect hepatosplenomegaly, pleural effusion, and ascites which may be associated with elevated vascular endothelial growth factor (VEGF).

Further routine laboratory investigations are focused especially on hematopoietic and immune systems to identify changes in platelet counts and anemia. Markers for acute phase response, such as serum C-reactive protein (CRP), ferritin, and IL-6, are important markers of the disease when present. Measurement of IL-6 is especially important because it is one of the therapeutic targets. Other investigations are focused on identifying associated conditions as well as organ changes associated with CD, such as autoimmune conditions or neuropathy.

UNICENTRIC CASTLEMAN DISEASE

UCD was the first subtype of CD to be described and is now well characterized even though its cause remains unknown. UCD can be observed in adults but classically affects young adults or children. UCD is featured with local lymph node enlargement or a solitary mass, with few general symptoms in most cases. No symptoms are present in approximately 60% of the cases, and it is not uncommon that the diagnosis is performed fortuitously.[4] The main manifestation of UCD can be related to local complications of a mass or lymph node enlargement with extrinsic compression. Renal obstruction, dyspnea, cough, abdominal pain, and other signs have been reported.[6] Pathology examination reveals a hyaline-vascular type in 70% of cases, a plasma cell type in 10% to 20% of the cases, or rarely, a mixed form.[5] Patients with the

Table 2
Standard investigative workup in Castleman disease (following lymph node biopsy)

Recommended Initial Investigative Workup at	Expected Results
Radiological investigation: PET-CT (preferred) or CT of neck, chest, abdomen, and pelvis	Differentiate UCD from MCD and assess disease activity (standardized uptake value between 2.5 and 5)
Complete blood count: Hemoglobin, platelet count	Anemia, thrombocytosis (or thrombocytopenia in TAFRO or ITP)
Serum chemistry: Total protein, albumin, globulin, LDH	Elevated total proteins, hypoalbuminemia, hyperglobulinemia, elevated LDH
Protein electrophoresis, immunofixation, and quantitative immunoglobulin	Polyclonal hypergammaglobulinemia, negative immunofixation, polyclonal elevation of one or more classes (IgG, IgA, IgM) of immunoglobulins, no monoclonal spike
Markers of inflammation	Elevated erythrocyte sedimentation rate, CRP, serum ferritin, and fibrinogen
Serum cytokine levels: IL6 and in select cases VEGF	Elevated IL6 (not all cases in UCD), elevated VEGF in select patients
Serologic investigations for associated conditions	
Viral serology for HHV8, HIV	If positive, recommend quantitative assay and staining of lymph node biopsy for HHV8; more common in plasmacytic and mixed variant
Serologic investigations for autoimmune disorders, if clinically suspected	ANA and others; depending upon involved organ, positive results may be observed
IgH gene rearrangement study on lymph node specimen	Rule out clonal disorder, mainly occult lymphoma
Nerve conduction studies as indicated	In cases with symptoms of neuropathy

hyaline-vascular type often present no systemic symptoms and an intrathoracic lesion, whereas patients with the plasma cell type have more often an extrathoracic lesion and systemic symptoms, with biological abnormalities, mainly anemia, and hypergammaglobulinemia. An important complication associated with UCD, often in the younger age group, is pemphigus vulgaris or paraneoplastic pemphigus that could be potentially extremely severe and life threatening when associated with pulmonary involvement (see later discussion).[8] Other clinical manifestations could include peripheral neuropathy and rarely autoimmune cytopenia. Radiographs and CT scan help to confirm the unique location of the lesion and can often reveal the presence of calcification and highly vascularized lesions.[9] MRI and PET scans are also useful to evaluate the extent of the lesion and to identify small lesions featured by an increased metabolic activity.[9] Few or no biological abnormalities are present in general, but elevated CRP and hypergammaglobulinemia can be observed mainly in the plasmacytic variant. Both histologic types (hyaline vascular and plasmacytic type) are treated by excision, and systemic abnormalities associated with the plasma cell type resolve with excision.[10] The main differential diagnoses of UCD are lymphoma, solid tumors, follicular hyperplasia, and toxoplasma lymphadenitis.

As opposed to UCD, MCD is featured by important and often severe systemic symptoms that are mainly related to the release of various cytokines, including IL-6 and IL-10. Two distinct MCD have been well characterized to date: HHV8-related

MCD and iMCD. The main clinical and paraclinical features of UCD and MCD are reported in **Table 3**, and a simplified algorithm is provided to illustrate CD diagnosis in **Fig. 1**.

HUMAN HERPESVIRUS 8 AND HUMAN IMMUNODEFICIENCY VIRUS-POSITIVE MULTICENTRIC CASTLEMAN DISEASE

HHV8 and HIV-positive multicentric Castleman disease corresponds to the most frequent form of MCD. Its incidence has increased over the time with the advent of antiretroviral therapies.[11] General symptoms are important and include high fever and asthenia in more than 90% of the cases, splenomegaly, peripheral lymphadenopathy, edema, and cough. Biologically, anemia, thrombocytopenia, hypoalbuminemia, and elevated CRP levels are common. Positive direct antiglobulin test and autoimmune hemolytic anemia (AIHA) are present in 30% to 40% of the cases. Hemophagocytic lymphohistiocytosis is not uncommon. Active HHV8 infection is always present, and viral load is useful to monitor the disease activity. Conversely, there is no correlation between HIV viral load or CD4 count and MCD.[2] Kaposi sarcoma can coexist with MCD, and cutaneous and mucous lesions must be detected. Lymph node biopsy reveals the presence of large plasmablasts (also named immunoblasts), usually immunoglobulin M (IgM) λ restricted, within mantle zones of involved lymph nodes corresponding to HHV8-infected cells and latent nuclear antigen-1 (LANA-1) positive staining, with a plasma cell or a mixed form subtype.[12] Plasmablasts may coalesce and be identified as "microlymphoma," although no lymphoma is present. Kaposi sarcoma lesions can coexist with CD in up to 40% of the cases. Two important specificities are related to this setting, the risk of Kaposi sarcoma exacerbation and the risk of plasmablastic lymphoma. The latter can occur later after the MCD diagnosis or can be present at the diagnosis, and a careful pathology evaluation should be done. Clonality evaluation might be helpful to rule out the presence of a true lymphoma. The disease is in the vast majority responsive to rituximab-based regimen and etoposide that has greatly improved the prognosis and the outcome, and decreased the risk of plasmablastic lymphoma.[13] However, relapse can occur, and follow-up is necessary.

MULTICENTRIC CASTLEMAN DISEASE HUMAN HERPESVIRUS 8-POSITIVE HUMAN IMMUNODEFICIENCY VIRUS-NEGATIVE

A subset of HHV8-related MCD affects HIV-negative patients. The clinical presentation is similar to HIV-positive MCD, with important systemic symptoms, asymmetric lymphadenopathy, and splenomegaly. High CRP level, hypoalbuminemia, hypergammaglobulinemia, positive Direct antiglobulin (Coombs) test (DAT), and hemophagocytic lymphohistiocytosis are not uncommon. HHV8 viral load is high, and the virus can be detected in the lymph nodes with LANA-1 staining in addition to the classical findings of MCD (depleted germinal centers, expanded mantle zones, prominent infiltration of plasma cells in the interfollicular region, and vascular hyperplasia). The presence of Kaposi sarcoma is also frequent as well as the increased risk of HHV8-related lymphoma. The disease is sensitive and responsive to rituximab and etoposide-based regimen but relapse is frequent and requires a close monitoring.

IDIOPATHIC MULTICENTRIC CASTLEMAN DISEASE

iMCD is featured by systemic signs, lymphadenopathy at multiple locations, and typical histologic findings of CD. Autoimmunity-related symptoms, including arthritis and renal dysfunction with proteinuria, are more often observed in iMCD than in

Table 3
Main clinical and paraclinical characteristics of the different subtypes of Castleman disease

	UCD (n = 43)	HHV8+ HIV+ MCD (n = 61)	HHV8+ HIV− MCD (n = 18)	iMCD (n = 31)
Clinical signs				
Fever, %	7	~100	~100	13 to 52
Lymphadenopathy	Localized	Diffuse	Diffuse	Diffuse
Hepatomegaly or Splenomegaly, %	2	95	72	19
Pleural effusion/ascites, %	No	18	NA	13
Respiratory symptoms, %	2	61	17	13
Paraclinical				
Anemia or AIHA, %	12.5	43	33	40
Thrombocytopenia, %	No	33	11	17
Hypoalbuminemia, %	5	70	61	17
PET-CT	Positive, localized	Positive, multiple	Positive, multiple	Positive, multiple

Data from Refs.[2–4]

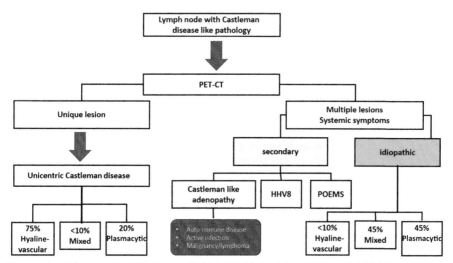

Fig. 1. Algorithm to assess CD diagnosis. (*Adapted from* Fajgenbaum DC, Uldrick TS, Bagg A, et al. International, evidence-based consensus diagnostic criteria for HHV-8-negative/idiopathic multicentric Castleman disease. Blood 2017;129(12):1651; with permission.)

HHV8-related MCD or UCD. In the lymph nodes, a distinct immunophenotype of the lymphocytes with higher numbers of CD3[+] lymphocytes and lower frequency of CD19[+]/CD5[+] have been reported in iMCD patients compared with UCD patients.[4] In addition, the absence of HHV8 leads to no association with Kaposi sarcoma or increased risk of plasmablastic lymphoma. Because the clinical presentation could overlap with the clinical presentation of other diseases, it is extremely important to rule out other differential diagnoses, including lymphoma, autoimmune lymphoproliferative syndrome, rheumatoid arthritis, systemic lupus, and active infections (HIV, tuberculosis, Epstein-Barr virus). PET/CT scan is useful to identify involved lymph nodes and to monitor the disease. Recently, consensus diagnostic criteria have been published and are reported in **Table 4**.[14]

SPECIFIC PRESENTATIONS OF CASTLEMAN DISEASE
Paraneoplastic Pemphigus

Paraneoplastic pemphigus corresponds to the clinical presentation of pemphigus vulgaris in the context of a malignancy, mainly B-cell malignancy.[15] In CD, the presence of mouth ulceration is highly suggestive of pemphigus and requires a careful skin and pulmonary evaluation. The severity of the disease directly correlates with involvement of the lung. Pulmonary manifestations include dyspnea, hypoxemia, obliterans bronchiolitis, and obstructive pulmonary ventilatory dysfunction.[8] No specific histology of CD is associated with the occurrence of paraneoplastic pemphigus, but it is more frequent in the context of UCD. Autoantibodies targeting desmoplakin are often present.[16] Steroids may be used with relative success, although the best treatment remains the surgical excision of CD lesions.

POEMS

POEMS syndrome refers to the presence of Peripheral neuropathy, Organomegaly, Endocrinopathy, Monoclonal gammopathy, and Skin changes. Other clinical findings are also frequently observed in that setting, including papilledema, pleural effusions,

Table 4
Consensus diagnostic criteria for idiopathic multicentric Castleman disease

Major criteria	
Histology	Regressed/atrophic germinal centers (grade >2) with expanded mantle zones composed of concentric rings ("onion skin" appearance)
	Follicular dendritic cells prominence
	Hypervascularity with prominent endothelium in the interfollicular space and vessels penetrating into germinal centers ("lollipop" appearance)
	Sheetlike and polytypic plasmacytosis in the interfollicular space (grade >2)
	Presence of hyperplastic germinal centers
Enlarged lymph nodes	2 lymph nodes with a short diameter >2 cm
Minor criteria	
Clinical	B symptoms
	Hepatomegaly or splenomegaly
	Fluid accumulation
	Lymphocytic interstitial pneumonitis
	Eruptive cherry hemangiomatosis or violaceous papules
Laboratory	Inflammatory syndrome: elevated CRP and hypoalbuminemia
	Anemia
	Thrombocytopenia or thrombocytosis
	Proteinuria
	Polyclonal hypergammaglobulinemia
Exclusion criteria	
Active or uncontrolled infection (HHV8, HIV, toxoplasmosis, EBV, CMV)	
Autoimmune or autoinflammatory diseases (systemic lupus erythematous, rheumatoid arthritis, adult-onset Still disease, juvenile idiopathic arthritis, autoimmune lymphoproliferative syndrome)	
Malignancy (lymphoma, multiple myeloma, plasmacytoma, follicular dendritic cell sarcoma, POEMS syndrome)	

The diagnosis of iMCD is made if 2 major criteria and ≥2 minor criteria are present.
Adapted from Faigenbaum DC, Uldrick TS, Bagg A, et al. International, evidence-based consensus diagnostic criteria for HHV-8-negative/idiopathic multicentric Castleman disease. Blood 2017;129(12):1652; with permission.

ascites, sclerotic bone lesions, and thrombocytosis. Enlarged lymph nodes are often observed with CD like histology in up to 40% of the cases.[17] The isotype of the monoclonal gammopathy is almost exclusively λ with restricted usage of immunoglobulin λ light chain variable region. Bone marrow often shows megakaryocytic hyperplasia. The physiopathology of POEMS is poorly understood, but cytokines, including IL-6, IL-12, and VEGF, play an important role.[18,19]

TAFRO

The recently described TAFRO syndrome corresponds to a subtype of iMCD featured by thrombocytopenia (T), anasarca (A), fever (F), reticulin fibrosis (R), and organomegaly (O).[20] The presence of thrombocytopenia and the absence of hypergammaglobulinemia are particularly suggestive of TAFRO syndrome as compared with classic iMCD presentation. Lymph node pathology is featured by the classic CD findings with higher frequency of mixed subtype and hypervascular features. Outcome of this subgroup may be worse than other iMCD, but no specific mechanism or treatment has been identified to date for this specific subgroup.[21]

HEMOPHAGOCYTIC LYMPHOHISTIOCYTOSIS

MCD and especially HHV8-related MCD presentation can be featured by hemophagocytic lymphohistiocytosis as the initial presentation or at relapse.[3,22] In addition to the classic and above-described clinical symptoms of MCD, the patients present hypofibrinogenemia, elevated low-density lipoprotein (LDH) and triglycerides, and hemodynamic and potentially multiorgan failure. In that context, rapid diagnosis, including lymph node biopsy and treatment, is critical. Initial treatment with etoposide or vinblastine is very efficient. In the absence of efficacy and especially in the context of HHV8 and HIV-positive MCD, a diagnosis of plasmablastic or other lymphoma must be considered and other investigations should be performed.

AUTOIMMUNE CYTOPENIA

In the context of hypergammaglobulinemia, the direct antiglobulin test can be positive for IgG or IgG and complement without any biological hemolysis. However, AIHA is a relatively frequent complication of MCD present in up to 40% and can be the initial presentation of MCD. Immune thrombocytopenia (ITP) is less frequent but has been reported in 5% to 20% of MCD cases.[2,3,8] The combination of AIHA and ITP (Evans syndrome) in the context of CD requires ruling out diagnosis of autoimmune lymphoproliferative disorder. This latter is secondary to genetic alterations of FAS/FAS-ligand and can be featured by autoimmune cytopenia and Castleman-like lymph nodes. The detection of double-negative T-cell population (CD4$^-$ and CD8$^-$) is helpful to make the diagnosis.[23,24]

PERIPHERAL NEUROPATHY

Demyelinating peripheral neuropathy is frequently observed with CD. The pathophysiology is unknown, and there is no clear association between the severity of the peripheral neuropathy and the subtype of CD. In UCD, the peripheral neuropathy is less frequent, usually sensory, whereas in the context of MCD, the neuropathy can be more severe and sensorimotor. Any clinical evidence of peripheral neuropathy requires careful consideration of the diagnosis of POEMS syndrome.[25]

RENAL INVOLVEMENT

Renal alterations are frequently observed in MCD mainly in the plasma cell and mixed subtype. Two retrospective studies have reported renal abnormalities in up to 25% of MCD. Glomerular lesions, AA amyloidosis, and interstitial nephritis are the most common renal pathology findings. Lesions of thrombotic microangiopathy are the most frequent and can be observed in the presence of anti-ADAMTS13 antibodies.[26] Usually, adapted treatment of MCD, including chemotherapy, leads to renal remission.[27,28]

DIFFERENTIAL DIAGNOSIS

The presence of CD features on a lymph node biopsy is not sufficient to diagnose CD, and multiple diseases have been reported to be associated with Castleman-like changes in lymph nodes. The differential diagnosis of UCD includes other disorders that can present with an enlarged lymph node, mainly toxoplasma lymphadenitis, follicular hyperplasia, Hodgkin lymphoma, plasmacytoma, and often what is reported as reactive change. The differential diagnosis of MCD is a B-cell malignancy, mainly multiple myeloma, or non-Hodgkin lymphoma or Hodgkin lymphoma, and autoimmune connective disorder (rheumatoid arthritis and systemic lupus erythematous) that can present with CD-like adenopathy.[29,30]

In conclusion, CD is a heterogeneous entity with very diverse clinical presentation and outcome. Each subtype must be identified and treated per the specific complications. Extended and careful investigation is required to rule out differential diagnosis.

REFERENCES

1. Castleman B, Iverson L, Menendez VP. Localized mediastinal lymph node hyperplasia resembling thymoma. Cancer 1956;9(4):822–30.
2. Bower M, Newsom-Davis T, Naresh K, et al. Clinical features and outcome in HIV-associated multicentric Castleman's disease. J Clin Oncol 2011;29(18):2481–6.
3. Dossier A, Meignin V, Fieschi C, et al. Human herpesvirus 8-related Castleman disease in the absence of HIV infection. Clin Infect Dis 2013;56(6):833–42.
4. Yu L, Tu M, Cortes J, et al. Clinical and pathological characteristics of HIV- and HHV-8-negative Castleman disease. Blood 2017;129(12):1658–68.
5. Keller AR, Hochholzer L, Castleman B. Hyaline-vascular and plasma-cell types of giant lymph node hyperplasia of the mediastinum and other locations. Cancer 1972;29(3):670–83.
6. Talat N, Belgaumkar AP, Schulte KM. Surgery in Castleman's disease: a systematic review of 404 published cases. Ann Surg 2012;255(4):677–84.
7. Oksenhendler E, Duarte M, Soulier J, et al. Multicentric Castleman's disease in HIV infection: a clinical and pathological study of 20 patients. AIDS 1996;10(1):61–7.
8. Dong Y, Wang M, Nong L, et al. Clinical and laboratory characterization of 114 cases of Castleman disease patients from a single centre: paraneoplastic pemphigus is an unfavourable prognostic factor. Br J Haematol 2015;169(6):834–42.
9. Hill AJ, Tirumani SH, Rosenthal MH, et al. Multimodality imaging and clinical features in Castleman disease: single institute experience in 30 patients. Br J Radiol 2015;88(1049):20140670.

10. van Rhee F, Stone K, Szmania S, et al. Castleman disease in the 21st century: an update on diagnosis, assessment, and therapy. Clin Adv Hematol Oncol 2010; 8(7):486–98.

11. Powles T, Stebbing J, Bazeos A, et al. The role of immune suppression and HHV-8 in the increasing incidence of HIV-associated multicentric Castleman's disease. Ann Oncol 2009;20(4):775–9.

12. Dupin N, Diss TL, Kellam P, et al. HHV-8 is associated with a plasmablastic variant of Castleman disease that is linked to HHV-8-positive plasmablastic lymphoma. Blood 2000;95(4):1406–12.

13. Gerard L, Michot JM, Burcheri S, et al. Rituximab decreases the risk of lymphoma in patients with HIV-associated multicentric Castleman disease. Blood 2012; 119(10):2228–33.

14. Fajgenbaum DC, Uldrick TS, Bagg A, et al. International, evidence-based consensus diagnostic criteria for HHV-8-negative/idiopathic multicentric Castleman disease. Blood 2017;129(12):1646–57.

15. Kaplan I, Hodak E, Ackerman L, et al. Neoplasms associated with paraneoplastic pemphigus: a review with emphasis on non-hematologic malignancy and oral mucosal manifestations. Oral Oncol 2004;40(6):553–62.

16. Anhalt GJ, Kim SC, Stanley JR, et al. Paraneoplastic pemphigus. An autoimmune mucocutaneous disease associated with neoplasia. N Engl J Med 1990;323(25): 1729–35.

17. Dispenzieri A. POEMS syndrome: 2017 update on diagnosis, risk stratification, and management. Am J Hematol 2017;92(8):814–29.

18. Royer B, Merlusca L, Abraham J, et al. Efficacy of lenalidomide in POEMS syndrome: a retrospective study of 20 patients. Am J Hematol 2013;88(3):207–12.

19. Jaccard A, Royer B, Bordessoule D, et al. High-dose therapy and autologous blood stem cell transplantation in POEMS syndrome. Blood 2002;99(8):3057–9.

20. Takai K, Nikkuni K, Shibuya H, et al. [Thrombocytopenia with mild bone marrow fibrosis accompanied by fever, pleural effusion, ascites and hepatosplenomegaly. Rinsho Ketsueki 2010;51(5):320–5 [in Japanese].

21. Iwaki N, Fajgenbaum DC, Nabel CS, et al. Clinicopathologic analysis of TAFRO syndrome demonstrates a distinct subtype of HHV-8-negative multicentric Castleman disease. Am J Hematol 2016;91(2):220–6.

22. Stebbing J, Ngan S, Ibrahim H, et al. The successful treatment of haemophagocytic syndrome in patients with human immunodeficiency virus-associated multicentric Castleman's disease. Clin Exp Immunol 2008;154(3):399–405.

23. Rieux-Laucat F, Le Deist F, Hivroz C, et al. Mutations in Fas associated with human lymphoproliferative syndrome and autoimmunity. Science 1995;268(5215): 1347–9.

24. Rao VK, Oliveira JB. How I treat autoimmune lymphoproliferative syndrome. Blood 2011;118(22):5741–51.

25. Naddaf E, Dispenzieri A, Mandrekar J, et al. Clinical spectrum of Castleman disease-associated neuropathy. Neurology 2016;87(23):2457–62.

26. London J, Boutboul D, Agbalika F, et al. Autoimmune thrombotic thrombocytopenic purpura associated with HHV8-related multicentric Castleman disease. Br J Haematol 2017;178(3):486–8.

27. Xu D, Lv J, Dong Y, et al. Renal involvement in a large cohort of Chinese patients with Castleman disease. Nephrol Dial Transplant 2012;27(Suppl 3):iii119–25.

28. El Karoui K, Vuiblet V, Dion D, et al. Renal involvement in Castleman disease. Nephrol Dial Transplant 2011;26(2):599–609.

29. Kojima M, Nakamura S, Itoh H, et al. Systemic lupus erythematosus (SLE) lymphadenopathy presenting with histopathologic features of Castleman' disease: a clinicopathologic study of five cases. Pathol Res Pract 1997;193(8):565–71.

30. Maheswaran PR, Ramsay AD, Norton AJ, et al. Hodgkin's disease presenting with the histological features of Castleman's disease. Histopathology 1991;18(3): 249–53.

Unicentric Castleman Disease

Raymond S.M. Wong, MBChB, MD

KEYWORDS

- Castleman disease • Unicentric • Hyaline vascular variant • Plasma cell variant
- Interleukin 6

KEY POINTS

- Unicentric Castleman disease (UCD) is a rare condition that typically manifests as a slow-growing lymph node at a single anatomic site.
- Most UCD patients have hyaline vascular histologic subtype and they do not have systemic symptoms.
- Approximately 10% to 25% of patients have plasma cell variant morphology that can be associated with constitutional symptoms and laboratory abnormalities, reflecting excess interleukin 6 secretion.
- UCD has a good prognosis and complete surgical resection is the optimal approach.
- In UCD patients who have inoperable lesions or refractory to surgical resection, radiotherapy or systemic therapy, such as rituximab or chemotherapy, can be effective.

INTRODUCTION

In 1954, Benjamin Castleman described a 40-year-old man who presented with many years of fever, weakness, and nonproductive cough and was found to have a large mediastinal mass at fluoroscopy.[1] On surgical excision, the pathology showed unusual lymphoproliferation, which was characterized by lymph node hyperplasia and follicles with hyalinized foci. This case, followed by a series with 12 additional patients, subsequently identified and reported by Dr Castleman, was what is now known as unicentric Castleman disease (UCD).[2]

UCD is characterized by involvement of a single lymph node region and typically demonstrates an indolent course with progressive enlargement of the lesion. Using 2 commercial claims databases, the incidence of UCD was estimated to be 15.9 to 19.1 cases per million person-years and this translates to an annual incidence of approximately 4900 to 6000 patients with UCD in the United States.[3] UCD can occur

Department of Medicine and Therapeutics, Sir Y.K. Pao Cancer Centre, Prince of Wales Hospital, The Chinese University of Hong Kong, 30-32 Ngan Shing Street, Shatin, New Territories, Hong Kong
E-mail address: raymondwong@cuhk.edu.hk

Hematol Oncol Clin N Am 32 (2018) 65–73
https://doi.org/10.1016/j.hoc.2017.09.006
0889-8588/18/© 2017 Elsevier Inc. All rights reserved.

hemonc.theclinics.com

at any age. Based on some large case series, the median age at presentation is 30 years to 34 years and the disease occurs equally in men and women.[4-7] There was no association with HIV or human herpesvirus 8 infection and epidemiologic risk factors have not been identified.[8,9] Most cases of UCD had hyaline vascular (HV)-type histology (74–91%) but plasma cell (PC)-type histology had also been reported (9–26%).[10-13]

CLINICAL MANIFESTATIONS

Patients with UCD can be asymptomatic and the condition is discovered incidentally on imaging for other medical conditions. Others may present with symptoms relating to enlarged lymph node's compression on surrounding structures.

From a systematic review of published cases, including 278 patients with UCD, mean size of affected lymph node was 5.5 cm, which is larger than that in patients with multicentric Castleman disease (MCD). Common sites of presentation include chest (29%), neck (23%), abdomen (21%), and retroperitoneum (17%) whereas lymph nodes at other sites, such as axilla, groin, and pelvis, may also be involved.[14] Rarely, UCD presents in unusual sites, such as the lungs, orbits, nasopharynx, spleen, or small bowel.[15-20]

Patients with UCD in the peripheral lymph nodes chains may present with nontender lymphadenopathy. Lesions in the chest may present with cough, dyspnea, chest discomfort, or hemoptysis. Lesions in the abdomen, pelvis, and retroperitoneum may cause abdominal or back discomfort.[9] Bowel and ureteric obstruction have rarely been reported.[15,21] It is uncommon for UCD patients with HV pathology to have systemic symptoms or laboratory abnormalities reflecting excess interleukin (IL)-6 secretion.[22] On the other hand, in patients with PC pathology, constitutional symptoms (eg, B symptoms) and laboratory abnormalities (eg, anemia, elevated erythrocyte sedimentation rate and/or C-reactive protein, hypergammaglobulinemia, and hypoalbuminemia) have been observed.[9,10,23]

Given the rarity of UCD and the nonspecific nature of the presenting features, the clinical presentation of lymphadenopathy may raise suspicion of lymphomas in many cases.[14,24-26] In other cases, tumors of the organs where the UCD lesions are located, infectious or inflammatory diseases may be the initial working diagnoses.[15,19,27] Histologic examination is the key to a correct diagnosis.

INVESTIGATIONS AND DIAGNOSIS

Castleman disease (CD) is usually suspected based on imaging findings. Various imaging modalities, including ultrasonography, CT, MRI, and/or PET, may discover the enlarged lymph nodes incidentally and they are commonly used to evaluate a patients with UCD.

Plain Radiographs

Chest radiograph is typically the first-line imaging modality in the evaluation of thoracic disease. Patients with thoracic UCD may manifest as a rounded solitary mediastinal, hilar or lung mass that may be complicated by pleural effusion.[6,13,28,29] Such lesions may mimic thymoma, lymphoma, neurogenic tumor, bronchial adenomas, or lung tumor.[13,28] Abdominal and pelvic UCD is usually not be visible on abdominal radiographs unless the lesions are massive or have calcification sufficient to be visible on radiographs.[28]

Computed Tomography

The typical appearance of UCD on CT is a solitary, well-circumscribed, enlarged lymph node or localized nodal masses.[11,29-33] On noncontrast CT, the nodes were typically hypodense to isodense to skeletal muscle.[11,33] Homogeneous intense contrast enhancement has been reported to be characteristic of UCD in the thorax and abdomen, reflecting the hypervascularity of the lesion.[28,30,31] On double-phase CT scans, UCD has been reported to demonstrate mild enhancement at the arterial phase, and gradually uniform enhancement at venous phase.[33] Prominent feeding vessels may occasionally be seen.[28] In a case series evaluating the CT findings of 20 patients with UCD in the thorax, 3 patterns of involvement have been observed in patients with HV type UCD: a solitary, noninvasive mass (50% of cases); a dominant infiltrative mass with associated lymphadenopathy (40% of cases); or matted lymph-adenopathy without a dominant mass (10% of cases).[29] Meador and McLarney[34] reported that abdominal or pelvic tumors greater than 5 cm in diameter generally showed heterogeneous enhancement with low-attenuation areas consistent with ne-crosis or intralesional fibrosis. It has also been reported that lymph nodes in patients with HV variant enhanced more avidly than other histologic types[29,31] but other studies did not confirm the finding.[11,30]

Intralesional calcifications with a variety of patterns, including punctate, coarse, and arborizing (branching), have been reported, with punctate pattern the most com-mon.[11,28–31,34] The presence of absence of calcification did not correlate with any spe-cific subtype of CD.[11] The presence of calcification seen in CD, however, may help in differentiating CD from lymphoma, because calcification is rare in untreated lymphoma.[11]

MRI

MRI is useful in the evaluation of UCD. It can show the extent of the tumor and clarify the relationship to the adjacent structure with its excellent soft tissue contrast.[28] Most lesions are isointense or slightly hyperintense relative to skeletal muscle on T1-weighted images and hyperintense on T2-weighted images, reflecting the vascularity of the masses.[11,28,29,31,33,35,36] MRI can also demonstrate the feeding vessels as flow void structures.[28] Central linear hypointense septate may be seen and has been sug-gested to represent lamellar fibrosis.[35] Evaluation of calcification is limited, however, by MRI.[31]

Ultrasonography

Ultrasonography has been used to evaluate peripheral, abdominal, or pelvic lesions. Most lesions appear as nonspecific, well-defined hypoechoic masses without necro-sis on ultrasonography.[11,28,37] Prominent peripheral vessels around the mass can be seen and penetrating feeding vessels may be demonstrated on Doppler study.[28,37] Posterior acoustic enhancement of involved nodes has been reported.[11] The appear-ance of CD on ultrasonography may mimic lymphoma.

PET

PET provides information regarding the metabolic status of lymph node. Fludeoxyglu-cose F 18 (^{18}F-FDG) avid lesion has been demonstrated in patients with UCD.[10,11,38–41] In general, ^{18}F-FDG uptake is moderately increased in UCD lesions and the standardized uptake values are less than that observed in patients with lym-phoma. PET may help to localize small lesions, which may otherwise be difficult to di-agnose.[40] In addition, ^{18}F-FDG–PET/CT can detect abnormal uptake in nonenlarged lymph node and is more sensitive than contrast-enhanced CT in the evaluation and monitoring of CD.[35,38,42]

Laboratory Studies

A majority of patients with HV UCD do not have significant laboratory abnormalities. Many patients with PC pathology may show anemia, elevated erythrocyte sedimentation rate, and/or C-reactive protein, hypergammaglobulinemia, and hypoalbuminemia. It is difficult to achieve a definitive diagnosis by imaging or biochemical tests. Histologic examination is mandatory for confirming the diagnosis. The gold standard for diagnosis is an excisional biopsy from the lymph node. Fine needle aspiration is usually nondiagnostic.

TREATMENT
Surgery

Surgery provides a tissue-based diagnosis and cure of the condition if the lesion is amenable to complete resection. Complete surgical resection as the sole treatment modality is the preferred treatment of UCD.[14] The surgical approach in UCD should aim for complete resection of the primarily involved lymph node with free resection margins whereas locoregional systematic lymphadenectomy should be performed if a cluster of lymph nodes is involved. A visceral location of the dominant disease focus does not preclude a successful surgical approach.[14] Complete surgical excision can often eliminate systemic symptoms that are present.[43–45] Regional small "satellite" lymph nodes usually involute with surgical extirpation of the bulk of the disease.[22] Additional adenopathy in a new location has been reported to occur occasionally after a complete surgical resection.[10]

If complete surgical resection is not possible, for example, when the lesion involves vital structures, debulking surgery should be considered to reduce the local symptoms or compression on vital structures. Partial resection followed by clinical observation may result in lengthy remissions. Long-term follow-up is needed because recurrences have been reported to occur as late as 11 years after incomplete resection.[13,46] In addition, neoadjuvant therapy or embolization may be considered to reduce the size of the lesion and render it amenable to complete resection.[10,47,48] Preoperative embolization has also been reported to help minimize intraoperative bleeding.[49]

Radiotherapy

Local radiotherapy is a reasonable alternative treatment option for unresectable UCD. Chan and colleagues[8] reviewed 17 patients with UCD that were treated with radiotherapy alone, mostly with doses of 40 Gy to 45 Gy (range 27–60). Six patients achieved a complete response and 7 achieved a partial response. After median follow-up of 20 months (range 5–175), 3 patients had died, although only 1 of them was disease related.[8] Serious acute and late toxicities have been reported after radiotherapy for UCD.[50] Intensity modulated radiation therapy has been reported to offer a better treatment modality compared with conventional 3-D conformal techniques for patients with unresectable UCD involving the chest to reduce dose gradients and toxicity to the adjacent normal tissue.[51]

Other Therapeutic Options

For asymptomatic patients with low disease burden who cannot be treated with surgery or radiotherapy, watch and wait can be considered in view of the indolent nature of UCD.[9] Systemic therapeutic options for MCD, such as chemotherapy, rituximab, or anti–IL-6 therapy, can be considered for patients with UCD who are symptomatic but cannot be treated with surgery or radiotherapy or for those who fail to respond to such treatment.[9,10,47,52,53] Data of these treatments in UCD are limited, however, and the optimal treatment strategy is not well defined.

PROGNOSIS

Patients with UCD have excellent prognosis if complete resection can be done, which confers 10-year overall survival rates of more than 95%.[14] Long-term outcome of patients with UCD who underwent resective surgery was significantly better than for those who only had diagnostic surgery in a large case series.[14] Even in patients with unresectable UCD, limited available data suggested radiotherapy can offer good long-term response rate (overall survival of 82% at 20 months).[8] PC UCD has a worse prognosis then HV type.[5]

DISEASES ASSOCIATED WITH UNICENTRIC CASTLEMAN DISEASE
Paraneoplastic Pemphigus

UCD may occasionally be associated with paraneoplastic pemphigus, which is potentially life threatening.[7,54,55] Paraneoplastic pemphigus is an autoimmune condition that manifests as chronic mucocutaneous blistering, and the clinical lesions may resemble pemphigus, pemphigoid, erythema multiforme, graft-versus-host disease, or lichen planus.[54] All patients with paraneoplastic pemphigus have concomitant occurrence of either occult or confirmed systemic neoplasm. In a review including 163 cases of paraneoplastic pemphigus, approximately 18% of them had localized CD. Clinicians should consider UCD when signs and symptoms suggestive of paraneoplastic pemphigus are present in young patients.[9] Complete resection of UCD lesion usually results in complete remission or improvement of the mucocutaneous lesions.[9]

Lymphoma

Non-Hodgkin lymphoma (NHL) is more often associated with MCD but it has also been reported in patients with UCD. In a review of 8 patients with UCD associated with NHL, B-cell NHL occurred in 6 patients and NHL was found in the same area as UCD in less than 30% of cases.[25] NHL is usually diagnosed concurrently with CD or diagnosed after CD. On the other hand, Hodgkin disease has been reported more commonly associated with UCD than MCD.[25] The association occurs more commonly in patients with PC variant histology and an interfollicular variant of HD.[25,56] The prognosis of the association between HD and CD seems better than that for association between NHL and CD.[25]

Follicular Dendritic Cell Sarcoma

Follicular dendritic cell sarcoma is a rare malignancy.[57] Of the reported cases, 10% to 20% have been shown to be associated with UCD, mostly the HV type, which can be concurrent with or precede the sarcoma.[58–67] The sarcoma occurs more often in lymph nodes but extranodal sites can be involved. The most common presentation is intra-abdominal lesions. Complete surgical resection is the treatment of choice. The role of adjuvant chemotherapy and radiotherapy is not clear.[9,68]

SUMMARY

UCD is a rare condition of unknown etiology and typically presents as a solitary mass with a progressive enlargement and indolent course. UCD occurs with equal frequency in men and women and the median age of presentation is 30 years to 34 years. Patients with UCD can be asymptomatic or may have symptoms due to compression of adjacent structures. Approximately 75% to 90% of patients with UCD have HV histologic subtype whereas 10% to 25% patients have PC variant, which can be associated with constitutional symptoms and laboratory abnormalities, reflecting excess

IL-6 secretion. Imaging studies typically showed a solitary lesion, which may mimic a tumor. There is no reliable diagnostic method and its definitive diagnosis is based on histopathology report. The current standard of care of UCD is surgical, and complete resection of the mass is recommended, with high cure rate. If complete resection is not possible, radiation therapy can be considered. Systemic therapeutic options for MCD, such as chemotherapy, rituximab, or anti–IL-6 therapy, can be considered for patients with UCD who cannot be treated with surgery or radiotherapy or for those who fail to respond to such treatment. Patients with UCD have excellent prognosis especially with successful treatment.

REFERENCES

1. CASE records of the Massachusetts General Hospital Weekly Clinicopathological exercises: case 40011. N Engl J Med 1954;250(1):26–30.
2. Castleman B, Iverson L, Menendez VP. Localized mediastinal lymphnode hyperplasia resembling thymoma. Cancer 1956;9(4):822–30.
3. Munshi N, Mehra M, van de Velde H, et al. Use of a claims database to characterize and estimate the incidence rate for Castleman disease. Leuk Lymphoma 2015;56(5):1252–60.
4. Dispenzieri A, Armitage JO, Loe MJ, et al. The clinical spectrum of Castleman's disease. Am J Hematol 2012;87(11):997–1002.
5. Talat N, Schulte KM. Castleman's disease: systematic analysis of 416 patients from the literature. Oncologist 2011;16(9):1316–24.
6. Luo JM, Li S, Huang H, et al. Clinical spectrum of intrathoracic Castleman disease: a retrospective analysis of 48 cases in a single Chinese hospital. BMC Pulm Med 2015;15:34.
7. Dong Y, Wang M, Nong L, et al. Clinical and laboratory characterization of 114 cases of Castleman disease patients from a single centre: paraneoplastic pemphigus is an unfavourable prognostic factor. Br J Haematol 2015;169(6): 834–42.
8. Chan KL, Lade S, Prince HM, et al. Update and new approaches in the treatment of Castleman disease. J Blood Med 2016;7:145–58.
9. Soumerai JD, Sohani AR, Abramson JS. Diagnosis and management of Castleman disease. Cancer Control 2014;21(4):266–78.
10. Yu L, Tu M, Cortes J, et al. Clinical and pathological characteristics of HIV- and HHV-8-negative Castleman disease. Blood 2017;129(12):1658–68.
11. Hill AJ, Tirumani SH, Rosenthal MH, et al. Multimodality imaging and clinical features in Castleman disease: single institute experience in 30 patients. Br J Radiol 2015;88(1049):20140670.
12. Cronin DM, Warnke RA. Castleman disease: an update on classification and the spectrum of associated lesions. Adv Anat Pathol 2009;16(4):236–46.
13. Keller AR, Hochholzer L, Castleman B. Hyaline-vascular and plasma-cell types of giant lymph node hyperplasia of the mediastinum and other locations. Cancer 1972;29(3):670–83.
14. Talat N, Belgaumkar AP, Schulte KM. Surgery in Castleman's disease: a systematic review of 404 published cases. Ann Surg 2012;255(4):677–84.
15. Akram W, Degliuomini J, Wallack MK, et al. Unicentric Castleman's Disease masquerading as a carcinoid tumor of the small intestine. Am Surg 2016;82(9): 287–9.

16. Rawashdeh B, Meyer M, Yimin D, et al. Unicentric Castleman's disease presenting as a pulmonary mass: a diagnostic dilemma. Am J Case Rep 2015;16:259–61.

17. Lee HJ, Jeon HJ, Park SG, et al. Castleman's disease of the spleen. World J Gastroenterol 2015;21(5):1675–9.

18. Kang D, Lee J, Lee H, et al. Unicentric Castleman's disease in the orbit: a case report. Indian J Ophthalmol 2015;63(6):555–7.

19. Liu Y, Chen G, Qiu X, et al. Intrapulmonary unicentric Castleman disease mimicking peripheral pulmonary malignancy. Thorac Cancer 2014;5(6):576–80.

20. Tsai MH, Pai HH, Yen PT, et al. Nasopharyngeal Castleman's disease. J Formos Med Assoc 1996;95(11):877–80.

21. Genoni M, De Lorenzi D, Bogen M, et al. Castleman's disease. Dtsch Med Wochenschr 1993;118(37):1316–20 [in German].

22. van Rhee F, Stone K, Szmania S, et al. Castleman disease in the 21st century: an update on diagnosis, assessment, and therapy. Clin Adv Hematol Oncol 2010;8(7):486–98.

23. Casper C. The aetiology and management of Castleman disease at 50 years: translating pathophysiology to patient care. Br J Haematol 2005;129(1):3–17.

24. Martino G, Cariati S, Tintisona O, et al. Atypical lymphoproliferative disorders: Castleman's disease. Case report and review of the literature. Tumori 2004;90(3):352–5.

25. Larroche C, Cacoub P, Soulier J, et al. Castleman's disease and lymphoma: report of eight cases in HIV-negative patients and literature review. Am J Hematol 2002;69(2):119–26.

26. Zarate-Osorno A, Medeiros LJ, Danon AD, et al. Hodgkin's disease with coexistent Castleman-like histologic features. A report of three cases. Arch Pathol Lab Med 1994;118(3):270–4.

27. Ochoa-Escudero M, Herrera DA, Dublin AB, et al. Unicentric Castleman's disease in the posterior cervical space mimicking a schwannoma. Eur Ann Otorhinolaryngol Head Neck Dis 2016;133(3):191–3.

28. Ko SF, Hsieh MJ, Ng SH, et al. Imaging spectrum of Castleman's disease. AJR Am J Roentgenol 2004;182(3):769–75.

29. McAdams HP, Rosado-de-Christenson M, Fishback NF, et al. Castleman disease of the thorax: radiologic features with clinical and histopathologic correlation. Radiology 1998;209(1):221–8.

30. Kwon S, Lee KS, Ahn S, et al. Thoracic Castleman disease: computed tomography and clinical findings. J Comput Assist Tomogr 2013;37(1):1–8.

31. Bonekamp D, Horton KM, Hruban RH, et al. Castleman disease: the great mimic. Radiographics 2011;31(6):1793–807.

32. Kim TJ, Han JK, Kim YH, et al. Castleman disease of the abdomen: imaging spectrum and clinicopathologic correlations. J Comput Assist Tomogr 2001;25(2):207–14.

33. Jiang XH, Song HM, Liu QY, et al. Castleman disease of the neck: CT and MR imaging findings. Eur J Radiol 2014;83(11):2041–50.

34. Meador TL, McLarney JK. CT features of Castleman disease of the abdomen and pelvis. AJR Am J Roentgenol 2000;175(1):115–8.

35. Madan R, Chen JH, Trotman-Dickenson B, et al. The spectrum of Castleman's disease: mimics, radiologic pathologic correlation and role of imaging in patient management. Eur J Radiol 2012;81(1):123–31.

36. Ecklund K, Hartnell GG. Mediastinal Castleman disease: MR and MRA features. J Thorac Imaging 1994;9(3):156–9.

37. Konno K, Ishida H, Hamashima Y, et al. Color Doppler findings in Castleman's disease of the mesentery. J Clin Ultrasound 1998;26(9):474–8.
38. Lee ES, Paeng JC, Park CM, et al. Metabolic characteristics of Castleman disease on 18F-FDG PET in relation to clinical implication. Clin Nucl Med 2013; 38(5):339–42.
39. Li YM, Liu PH, Zhang YH, et al. Radiotherapy of unicentric mediastinal Castleman's disease. Chin J Cancer 2011;30(5):351–6.
40. Toita N, Kawamura N, Hatano N, et al. A 5-year-old boy with unicentric Castleman disease affecting the mesentery: utility of serum IL-6 level and (18)F-FDG PET for diagnosis. J Pediatr Hematol Oncol 2009;31(9):693–5.
41. Murphy SP, Nathan MA, Karwal MW. FDG-PET appearance of pelvic Castleman's disease. J Nucl Med 1997;38(8):1211–2.
42. Barker R, Kazmi F, Stebbing J, et al. FDG-PET/CT imaging in the management of HIV-associated multicentric Castleman's disease. Eur J Nucl Med Mol Imaging 2009;36(4):648–52.
43. Bejjani J, Lemieux B, Gariepy G, et al. Complete anemia reversal after surgical excision of mesenteric hyaline-vascular unicentric Castleman disease. Can J Surg 2009;52(5):E197–8.
44. Herrada J, Cabanillas F, Rice L, et al. The clinical behavior of localized and multicentric Castleman disease. Ann Intern Med 1998;128(8):657–62.
45. Yoshizaki K, Matsuda T, Nishimoto N, et al. Pathogenic significance of interleukin-6 (IL-6/BSF-2) in Castleman's disease. Blood 1989;74(4):1360–7.
46. Olscamp G, Weisbrod G, Sanders D, et al. Castleman disease: unusual manifestations of an unusual disorder. Radiology 1980;135(1):43–8.
47. Bandera B, Ainsworth C, Shikle J, et al. Treatment of unicentric Castleman disease with neoadjuvant rituximab. Chest 2010;138(5):1239–41.
48. Safford SD, Lagoo AS, Mahaffey SA. Preoperative embolization as an adjunct to the operative management of mediastinal Castleman disease. J Pediatr Surg 2003;38(9):E21–3.
49. Robert JH, Sgourdos G, Kritikos N, et al. Preoperative embolization of hypervascular Castleman's disease of the mediastinum. Cardiovasc Intervent Radiol 2008; 31(1):186–8.
50. Neuhof D, Debus J. Outcome and late complications of radiotherapy in patients with unicentric Castleman disease. Acta Oncol 2006;45(8):1126–31.
51. Matthiesen C, Ramgopal R, Seavey J, et al. Intensity modulated radiation therapy (IMRT) for the treatment of unicentric Castlemans disease: a case report and review of the use of radiotherapy in the literature. Radiol Oncol 2012;46(3):265–70.
52. Abid MB, Peck R, Abid MA, et al. Is tocilizumab a potential therapeutic option for refractory unicentric Castleman disease? Hematol Oncol 2017. [Epub ahead of print].
53. Uysal B, Demiral S, Gamsiz H, et al. Castleman's disease and radiotherapy: a single center experience. J Cancer Res Ther 2015;11(1):170–3.
54. Sehgal VN, Srivastava G. Paraneoplastic pemphigus/paraneoplastic autoimmune multiorgan syndrome. Int J Dermatol 2009;48(2):162–9.
55. Kaplan I, Hodak E, Ackerman L, et al. Neoplasms associated with paraneoplastic pemphigus: a review with emphasis on non-hematologic malignancy and oral mucosal manifestations. Oral Oncol 2004;40(6):553–62.
56. Filliatre-Clement L, Busby-Venner H, Moulin C, et al. Hodgkin Lymphoma and Castleman Disease: when one blood disease can hide another. Case Rep Hematol 2017;2017:9423205.

57. Monda L, Warnke R, Rosai J. A primary lymph node malignancy with features suggestive of dendritic reticulum cell differentiation. A report of 4 cases. Am J Pathol 1986;122(3):562–72.
58. Chan AC, Chan KW, Chan JK, et al. Development of follicular dendritic cell sarcoma in hyaline-vascular Castleman's disease of the nasopharynx: tracing its evolution by sequential biopsies. Histopathology 2001;38(6):510–8.
59. Lee IJ, Kim SC, Kim HS, et al. Paraneoplastic pemphigus associated with follicular dendritic cell sarcoma arising from Castleman's tumor. J Am Acad Dermatol 1999;40(2 Pt 2):294–7.
60. Fornelli A, Mureden A, Eusebi V. Follicular dendritic cell tumor and unusual vascular lesion in lymph node with Castleman's disease. Description of a case. Pathologica 1998;90(2):146–51 [in Italian].
61. Andriko JW, Kaldjian EP, Tsokos M, et al. Reticulum cell neoplasms of lymph nodes: a clinicopathologic study of 11 cases with recognition of a new subtype derived from fibroblastic reticular cells. Am J Surg Pathol 1998;22(9):1048–58.
62. Lin O, Frizzera G. Angiomyoid and follicular dendritic cell proliferative lesions in Castleman's disease of hyaline-vascular type: a study of 10 cases. Am J Surg Pathol 1997;21(11):1295–306.
63. Katano H, Kaneko K, Shimizu S, et al. Follicular dendritic cell sarcoma complicated by hyaline-vascular type Castleman's disease in a schizophrenic patient. Pathol Int 1997;47(10):703–6.
64. Chan JK, Fletcher CD, Nayler SJ, et al. Follicular dendritic cell sarcoma. Clinicopathologic analysis of 17 cases suggesting a malignant potential higher than currently recognized. Cancer 1997;79(2):294–313.
65. Lauritzen AF, Ralfkiaer E. Histiocytic sarcomas. Leuk Lymphoma 1995;18(1–2): 73–80.
66. Chan JK, Tsang WY, Ng CS, et al. Follicular dendritic cell tumors of the oral cavity. Am J Surg Pathol 1994;18(2):148–57.
67. Ruco LP, Gearing AJ, Pigott R, et al. Expression of ICAM-1, VCAM-1 and ELAM-1 in angiofollicular lymph node hyperplasia (Castleman's disease): evidence for dysplasia of follicular dendritic reticulum cells. Histopathology 1991;19(6):523–8.
68. Hwang SO, Lee TH, Bae SH, et al. Transformation of Castleman's disease into follicular dendritic cell sarcoma, presenting as an asymptomatic intra-abdominal mass. Korean J Gastroenterol 2013;62(2):131–4.

Treatment of Kaposi Sarcoma Herpesvirus– Associated Multicentric Castleman Disease

 CrossMark

Kathryn Lurain, MD, MPH, Robert Yarchoan, MD,
Thomas S. Uldrick, MD, MS*

KEYWORDS

- Kaposi sarcoma herpesvirus • Human herpesvirus-8
- Multicentric Castleman disease • Human interleukin-6 • Viral interleukin 6
- Rituximab • Liposomal doxorubicin

KEY POINTS

- Kaposi sarcoma herpesvirus (KSHV)-associated multicentric Castleman disease is a B-cell lymphoproliferative disorder caused by KSHV that is characterized by waxing and waning inflammatory symptoms, laboratory abnormalities, edema, adenopathy, and splenomegaly. It is most common in patients with HIV.
- Four weekly doses of rituximab, 375 mg/m^2, lead to remission in a majority of mildly symptomatic patients but may lead to exacerbation of concurrent Kaposi sarcoma (KS).
- Rituximab, 375 mg/m^2, plus liposomal doxorubicin, 20 mg/m^2, administered every 3 weeks effectively treats patients with aggressive disease or concurrent KS.
- Rituximab-based treatment has increased 5-year overall survival to more than 90%.
- Current studies are evaluating targeted rituximab-sparing approaches that may decrease toxicity and/or be appropriate for patients with concurrent KS.

INTRODUCTION

Castleman disease is a term used to describe a variety of pathologic entities ranging from indolent localized angiofollicular hyperplasia (unicentric Castleman disease), as first described by Benjamin Castleman in the 1950s, to multicentric lymphoproliferations associated with inflammatory symptoms (multicentric Castleman disease [MCD]). One epidemiologically distinct plasmablastic form of MCD described in

Disclosures: See last page of article.
HIV and AIDS Malignancy Branch, Center for Cancer Research, National Cancer Institute, 10 Center Drive, Bethesda, MD 20892-1868, USA
* Corresponding author. HIV and AIDS Malignancy Branch, Center for Cancer Research, NCI, 10 Center Drive 6N106, Bethesda, MD 20892-1868.
E-mail address: uldrickts@mail.nih.gov

patients with HIV and associated with high mortality[1] was found caused by a newly discovered virus, called Kaposi sarcoma–associated herpesvirus (KSHV) or human herpesvirus 8 (HHV-8). KSHV was first identified as the etiologic agent for Kaposi sarcoma (KS) and is now recognized as the cause of almost all MCD in HIV-positive patients and rare cases of MCD in HIV-negative patients.[2]

KSHV-MCD is clinically characterized by intermittent inflammatory symptoms, cytopenias, edema lymphadenopathy, and splenomegaly, which often wax and wane. The diagnosis is confirmed pathologically, generally through a lymph node biopsy. Disease manifestations are associated with elevated levels of cytokines, especially interleukin (IL)-6 and IL-10.[3–5] Untreated, KSHV-MCD is generally lethal within 2 years.[5] Its rarity, intermittent manifestations, association with HIV, and nonspecific symptoms make diagnosing KSHV-MCD a challenge. The past decade, however, has seen the development of several effective therapies and substantial improvement in overall survival; therefore, increased recognition and timely diagnosis are important.

EPIDEMIOLOGY

KSHV-MCD incidence is unknown and the disease is almost certainly underdiagnosed. Powles and colleagues[6] estimated the incidence of KSHV-MCD in HIV-positive individuals to be 4.3 cases per 10,000 person-years and noted increasing incidence despite availability of effective antiretroviral therapy (ART) for HIV. KSHV-MCD often occurs in the setting of suppressed HIV, relatively preserved $CD4^+$ T-cell counts, and evidence of KSHV-specific $CD8^+$ T-cell response.[7,8] An improved understanding of the timing of KSHV-MCD diagnosis in relation to initiation of ART is required. It is possible that like KS and lymphoma, incidence is highest in the first year after ART initiation.[9]

KSHV-MCD is especially likely to be underdiagnosed in areas of sub-Saharan Africa with a high seroprevalence of both KSHV and HIV.[10–12] Unlike developed countries where KSHV prevalence in the general population is 2% to 5%, KSHV is endemic in large parts of sub-Saharan African, with 40% to greater than 80% of adults seropositive in much of the region.[10,11] The lack of reported KSHV-MCD cases almost certainly represents underdiagnosis, because KSHV-MCD has been described among African immigrants.[13,14] Due to lack of pathology services in many parts of sub-Saharan Africa, KS is sometimes treated empirically and without evaluation for concurrent KSHV-MCD in suspected cases. Additionally, fevers and lymphadenopathy, when present, are often empirically treated as tuberculosis.[13,15] Increased diagnostic capacity for Kaposi sarcoma herpesvirus-associated diseases, including KSHV-MCD, is needed in this setting.

PATHOGENESIS

KSHV is a gammaherpesvirus, most closely related to Epstein-Barr virus, with latent and lytic phases characteristic of all herpesviruses. In addition to KSHV-MCD, it is the etiologic agent of KS, primary effusion lymphoma (PEL), and Kaposi sarcoma herpesvirus-associated diffuse large B-cell lymphoma. Also, it is the cause of a newly identified condition called KSHV inflammatory cytokine syndrome, in which patients have severe inflammatory symptoms that mimic KSHV-MCD but lack the requisite pathologic findings of KSHV-MCD.[16,17]

KSHV encodes several proteins that allow for immune evasion via down-regulation of surface proteins required for immune surveillance.[18,19] The development of KSHV-MCD in HIV-positive patients may be related to reduction or functional impairment of invariant natural killer T (iNKT) cells.[20] iNKT cells play a major role in innate immunity and control of EBV infected B cells through activation of glycolipid antigens presented by the major histocompatibiity complex class 1–related molecule, CD1d, as well as stimulating the expansion and maturation of other immune cells.[21] In vitro studies of human tonsillar B cells suggest KSHV-MCD pathogenesis begins with KSHV infection via oral transmission of tonsillar IgM λ–expressing B cells that proliferate into plasma-blasts characteristic of KSHV-MCD.[22]

Expression of latent and lytic genes varies among Kaposi sarcoma herpesvirus-associated disorders.[23] In KS and PEL, a majority of genes expressed are latent genes with lytic proteins expressed in only a minority of cells, although in PEL, a KSHV-encoded viral IL-6 (vIL-6) is sometimes expressed in the absence of other lytic genes. In KSHV-MCD, however, a substantial proportion of the KSHV-infected plasmablasts in affected lymph nodes express lytic proteins. In some cases, the full lytic repertoire is expressed, and in other cases only vIL-6 is expressed.[23–25] Excess human cytokines, namely human IL-6 (hIL-6), IL-10, tumor necrosis factor α, and IL-1, are also important in the pathogenesis of KSHV-MCD.[5,26,27] vIL-6 shares 25% homology with its human counterpart. Unlike hIL-6, it binds directly to and signals through glycoprotein (gp)130, allowing it to affect a broad range of cells.[28–30] By contrast, hIL-6 signaling requires binding of both the classic IL-6 receptor, gp80, as well its coreceptor, gp130, which is ubiquitously expressed. Similar to hIL-6, serum vIL-6 levels correlate with the symptoms and laboratory abnormalities associated with active disease.[26,31] Although v-IL6 is often considered a lytic gene, it may be specifically up-regulated in KSHV-MCD by X-box binding protein 1.[32] There is also evidence that vIL-6 itself activates hIL-6, further driving KSHV-MCD pathogenesis.[33] Additional protein products of latently expressed genes also play a role in the pathogenesis of KSHV-MCD, in particular viral FLICE-inhibitory protein, which has been shown to induce significant disturbances in serum cytokines and expansion of suppressed myeloid cells, allowing for host immune evasion, angiogenesis, and tumor progression in mouse models.[34]

DIAGNOSIS

KSHV-MCD should be suspected in patients with an appropriate combination of risk factors and constellation of clinical and laboratory findings (**Fig. 1**). Histopathologic

Clinical Suspicion
- **Clinical laboratories:** Complete blood cell count with differential, chemistries, albumin, immunoglobulins, CRP, HIV antibody (if HIV status unknown), HIV viral load, CD4+ T-cell count, KSHV viral load
- **Imaging:** CT neck, chest, abdomen, and pelvis; +/- ¹⁸FDG-PET

Pathological Evaluation
- **Lymph node biopsy** (excisional biopsy preferred)
- **Skin biopsy** (if cutaneous KS is suspected and not already confirmed)
- **Effusions** (cytopathology and flow cytometry to evaluate for PEL)

Diagnosis
- **KSHV-MCD**
- **KSHV-MCD + KS**
- **KSHV-MCD + PEL +/- KS**

Treatment & Monitoring
- **Asymptomatic KSHV-MCD** → Monitor every 1–3 mo with exam, labs, and KSHV viral load
- **Mildly symptomatic KSHV-MCD** → Weekly rituximab
- **Severely symptomatic KSHV-MCD** → Rituximab + liposomal doxorubicin/etoposide
- **KSHV-MCD + KS** → Rituximab + liposomal doxorubicin or clinical trial
- **MCD + PEL** → Treat for PEL

Fig. 1. Schema for the diagnosis and management of KSHV-MCD.

confirmation of the diagnosis by lymph node biopsy is required. Populations at highest risk include men who have sex with men and sub-Saharan Africans. Diagnosis requires a high level of suspicion on the part of the clinician because the features of KSHV-MCD overlap significantly with those seen in uncontrolled infections and lymphoid malignancies. Clinical features of KSHV-MCD include fatigue, fevers, night sweats, weight loss, volume overload (including ascites and pulmonary effusions), rashes, and nonspecific neurologic, sinus, respiratory, and gastrointestinal symptoms. The course may include relapsing and remitting symptoms. Many patients have concurrent KS and a clinician's suspicion for KSHV-MCD should be raised in patients with KS and the aforementioned symptoms and laboratory findings. CT classically shows diffuse lymphadenopathy and splenomegaly (**Fig. 2**A).[35] KSHV-MCD patients with active disease essentially always have an elevated C-reactive protein (CRP) and KSHV viral load.

Plasma or peripheral blood mononuclear cell measurements of KSHV viral load should be performed and monitored throughout the disease course because this correlates with active disease and response to treatment.[5] Patients may exhibit several other laboratory abnormalities during active disease, including cytopenias, hypoalbuminemia, hyponatremia, and elevated γ-globulin.[1,5,7] Biopsy confirmation of KS should be pursued if indicated, because concurrent KS has implications for the choice of KSHV-MCD treatment. All patients with KSHV-MCD should be tested for HIV.

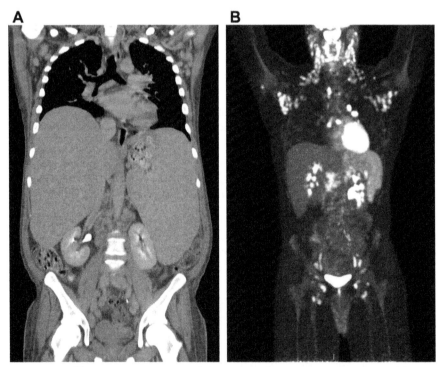

Fig. 2. CT and [18]FDG-PET in KSHV-MCD. (*A*) CT scans of an HIV-positive patient with KSHV-MCD prior to treatment showing hepatosplenomegaly and axillary and retroperitoneal adenopathy. (*B*) [18]FDG-PET of an HIV-positive patient with KSHV-MCD showing characteristic [18]FDG-avid cervical and axillary adenopathy as well as splenomegaly with diffuse increased [18]FDG uptake.

Although plasma levels of hIL-6 and IL-10 correlate with disease activity and response to treatment, these cytokines are not routinely followed outside of the scope of research activities.[5,27,36] Patients may become critically ill due to sepsis-like manifestations in the absence of infection driven by cytokine excess or exhibit pathologic and laboratory findings consistent with hemophagocytic syndrome.[37]

Histologically, KSHV-MCD–involved lymph nodes have expansion of KSHV-infected plasmablasts in the mantle zone of B-cell follicles. They also have reactive KSHV-uninfected plasmablasts. KSHV-infected plasmablasts may form microscopic collections, sometimes referred to as microlymphomas, although these are generally polyclonal.[38] KSHV-infected plasmablasts stain positive for Kaposi sarcoma herpesvirus-associated latent nuclear antigen-1 (LANA-1), and a proportion also express vIL-6. Unlike KSHV-associated germinotropic lymphoproliferative disorder and some cases of PEL, KSHV-MCD plasmablasts are negative for Epstein-Barr virus.[39,40] KSHV-infected plasmablasts express cytoplasmic IgM that is lambda light chain restricted but with a polyclonal pattern of immunoglobulin gene rearrangement (**Fig. 3**).[41] KS may be noted in the same lymph node (**Fig. 4**). A bone marrow biopsy is sometimes performed to evaluate cytopenias but is not required for diagnosis. In general, plasmacytosis is the predominant feature in the bone marrow with lymphoid aggregates and scattered KSHV-infected mononuclear cells less frequently seen.[42]

It is possible to diagnose KSHV-MCD from a lymph node core needle biopsy but an excisional lymph node biopsy is often required. In general, the most easily accessible enlarged lymph node should be chosen for pathologic evaluation. If an excisional lymph node biopsy, however, does not show KSHV-MCD and the diagnosis is strongly suspected, fludeoxyglucose F 18 (^{18}FDG)-PET scan should be performed. In KSHV-MCD, the most common findings are hypermetabolic symmetric ^{18}FDG-avid adenopathy with increased uptake notable in the spleen and bone marrow (see **Fig. 2**B).[35] Suspicious lymph nodes, which are often the largest and/or most ^{18}FDG avid, should be biopsied. Any effusions require cytopathologic examination. Effusions in KSHV-MCD may have elevated KSHV viral loads and show proliferation of polyclonal λ–restricted B cells; however, this finding has not been established as a method to definitively diagnose KSHV-MCD. More importantly, effusions should be examined to rule out PEL via cytopathology, flow cytometry, and B-cell clonality. In addition to PEL, patients with KSHV-MCD are at high risk of developing other non-Hodgkin lymphomas.[38,43,44]

TREATMENT

Although ART is generally insufficient for the treatment of KSHV-MCD, it is indicated for all patients with HIV. ART should be used concurrently along with KSHV-MCD–specific treatment in HIV-positive patients.[6,45] Patients with HIV-associated KSHV-MCD may obtain long remissions on ART with appropriate KSHV-MCD therapy. Although the effect of ART in preventing relapses is not proved, ART decreases mortality related to HIV.[46,47]

There is currently no Food and Drug Administration (FDA)-approved therapy for KSHV-MCD. Several cytotoxic chemotherapies with clinical activity in B-cell lymphomas have been used to treat KSHV-MCD, including etoposide, vincristine, vinblastine, cyclophosphamide, and doxorubicin.[1] Chemotherapy alone, however, is relatively ineffective. In 1 analysis between 1985 and 2006, the reported survival with these chemotherapies either alone or in combination was poor, with a median overall survival of 12 months. Major improvement in treatment responses and survival, however, came with the development of rituximab, a humanized monoclonal antibody against CD20 antigen on B cells.

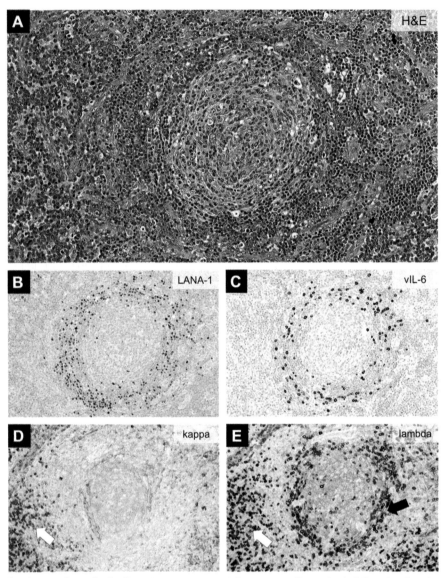

Fig. 3. Lymph node findings in KSHV-MCD. (*A*) Hematoxylin-eosin (H&E) stain showing typical features of Kaposi sarcoma herpesvirus-associated MCD. The involved lymph nodes have a regressed germinal center surrounded by layered mantle cells, vascular proliferation and hyalinization, and plasmacytosis in the interfollicular regions. (*B*) LANA-1 immunohisto-chemistry highlighting KSHV-infected plasmablasts residing in the mantle cell layers. (*C*) vIL-6 immunohistochemistry showing vIL-6 in a proportion of KSHV-infected plasmablasts. (*D, E*) Kappa and lambda light chain immunohistochemistry showing restricted lambda expression in the KSHV-infected plasmablasts (*black arrow*), while the interfollicular plasma cells are polytypic (*white arrows*).

Three prospective treatment studies and several cohort studies all show a substantial treatment effect of rituximab in KSHV-MCD. It is interesting that rituximab is effective despite that proliferating KSHV-infected B cells in KSHV-MCD are usually CD20$^-$.

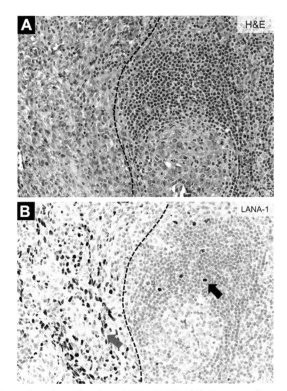

Fig. 4. Concominant lymph node KS and KSHV-MCD. (A) Hematoxylin-eosin stain demonstrating concomitant KS (*left of the dotted line*) and MCD (*right of the dotted line*). (B) LANA-1 immunohistochemistry highlighting the KSHV-infected cells. Note the different cytomorphology of KS cells (*red arrow*) and the plasmablasts in MCD (*black arrow*).

This may be because KSHV-uninfected CD20$^+$ B cells within the microenvironment secrete inflammatory cytokines and also serve as a major potential reservoir of KSHV infection and replication.[41] Two prospective phase 2 studies published in 2007 established the efficacy of rituximab in KSHV-MCD.[48,49] In the CastlemaB Trial, 24 patients with chemotherapy-dependent HIV-associated KSHV-MCD were administered 4 weekly infusions of rituximab (375 mg/m^2) after the discontinuation of chemotherapy. Overall survival was 92%, and 71% remained in remission at 1 year. A common problem was exacerbation of KS, noted in 8 of 12 patients with a previous diagnosis of KS despite the use of ART.[49] Bower and colleagues[48] reported similar results in 21 previously untreated patients with symptomatic HIV-associated KSHV-MCD treated with 4 weekly doses of rituximab (375 mg/m^2). At 2 years, overall survival was 95% and disease-free survival was 79%. More than one-third of the patients, however, had progression of KS.

To address the issue of KS exacerbation with the use of rituximab, a prospective trial evaluated the treatment of HIV-associated KSHV-MCD with a combination of rituximab, 375 mg/m^2, and liposomal doxorubicin, 20 mg/m^2, an FDA-approved KS therapy, every 3 weeks for a median of 4 cycles. Another potential advantage of concurrent use of liposomal doxubicin is that it can potentially target KSHV-MCD plasmablasts. Twelve of the 17 patients treated had concurrent KS. Exacerbation of KS was seen in only 1 patient, and KS regressed in most patients. The 3-year overall survival with this combination regimen was 81% and the event-free survival was 69%.[14] Rituximab also seems an effective therapy for KSHV-MCD in HIV-uninfected patients.[50] Infusion reactions that include rigors and fevers are common during the first administration of rituximab and may be due to a cytokine release syndrome. Premedication with steroids and diphenhydramine, as well as slow infusion rates during the first cycle, are warranted. When infusion reactions do occur, they are generally short lived and can be managed with meperidine. Infusions can be resumed at slower rates after resolution of symptoms. Although linked to exacerbation of KS, treatment with rituximab is associated with a substantially lower risk of non-Hodgkin lymphoma in KSHV-MCD patients.[44]

Antiherpesvirus therapy has also been evaluated in KSHV-MCD. Remissions have been described with the use of ganciclovir in 1 small retrospective study.[51] Two KSHV lytic genes, ORF36 and ORF21, encode enzymes that can phosphorylate ganciclovir and zidovudine (AZT), respectively, leading to accumulation of triphosphate moieties, which are toxic to KSHV-infected cells. Because of the role of viral enzymes in drug activation, non-KSHV–infected cells are spared.[52] Based on the principle of "virus activated cytotoxic therapy," a pilot study showed activity of high-dose AZT (600 mg orally every 6 hours) and valganciclovir (900 mg orally every 12 hours) in HIV-positive KSHV-MCD patients. Twelve of 14 patients achieved major clinical benefit with an 86% overall survival at 4 years. The median progression-free survival, however, was only 6 months. Although rituximab-based therapy is generally the treatment of choice, high-dose AZT and valganciclovir may be a useful alternative for patients with mild disease or who cannot tolerate rituximab.[53]

The authors follow a risk-stratified approach to treatment of KSHV-MCD, which takes into account the presence of concurrent KS or severe symptoms (see **Fig. 1**; **Table 1**). In patients with mild symptoms and laboratory abnormalities, 4 weekly doses of rituximab are generally sufficient to induce clinical remission in the vast majority of patients. Several case series have reported failure of rituximab in patients with aggressive disease, poor performance status, and organ failure.[54,55] Therefore, in patients with severe symptoms or a concurrent diagnosis of KS, the authors usually treat patients with rituximab combined with liposomal doxorubicin every 3 weeks.[14] More frequent initial rituximab dosing, that is, weekly during the first cycle, in combination with liposomal doxorubicin may also be appropriate. Excellent results of weekly rituximab combined with etoposide, 100 mg/m^2, for KSHV-MCD patients with severe symptoms have also been described, although etoposide is a less effective drug for treating KS.[56] In the rituximab era, combination chemotherapy does not have a role in treating KSHV-MCD except in the setting of concurrent lymphoma.

Treatment of KSHV-MCD should be individualized. The initiation of KSHV-MCD therapy should not be based on abnormal radiographic findings alone but instead on symptoms and abnormal laboratory findings. Duration of therapy should also be symptom based. There are no consensus guidelines for treatment response in KSHV-MCD. The CastlemaB Trial defined criteria for an MCD attack warranting treatment as the presence of fever, elevated CRP, and 3 clinical symptoms. The National Cancer Institute (NCI) criteria for treatment include at least 1 clinical symptom; the presence of anemia, thrombocytopenia, or hypoalbuminemia; and an elevated CRP.[53] The authors generally treat until resolution of clinical symptoms and significant improvement in these marker laboratory abnormalities. Like KSHV-MCD treatment, there is no standardized approach for patient follow-up. The authors generally see patients in clinic and measure their KSHV viral load every 3 months for the first year after therapy and less frequently thereafter. Patients with a persistently elevated KSHV viral load or residual adenopathy or splenomegaly are at higher risk of relapse and may

Table 1
Treatments for Kaposi sarcoma herpesvirus–associated multicentric Castleman disease

Therapy	Dose	Mechanism of Action	When to Use
Rituximab	375 mg/m^2 weekly ×4 wk	Depletes IL-6–secreting CD20$^+$ B cells	Mild symptomatic disease
Rituximab + liposomal doxorubicin	Rituximab 375 mg/m^2 + liposomal doxorubicin 20 mg/m^2 every 3 wk until response plateau	Addition of cytotoxic chemotherapy to treat CD20$^-$ MCD plasmablasts and KS spindle cells	Aggressive disease and/or concurrent KS
Rituximab + etoposide	Rituximab 375 mg/m^2 + etoposide 100 mg/m^2 IV weekly ×4 wk	Addition of cytotoxic chemotherapy to treat CD20$^-$ MCD plasmablasts	Aggressive disease
AZT + valganciclovir	Zidovidine 600 mg PO every 6 h + valganciclovir 900 mg PO every 12 h, d 1–7 of 21-d cycle	Virus-activated cytotoxic therapy	Mild disease with concurrent KS and/or patients allergic to rituximab

require more frequent monitoring, although the authors generally do not treat patients with these findings in the absence of symptoms and laboratory abnormalities.[57] Although consolidation or maintenance therapy have been used in the past, there is no clear role for these approaches. A recent study of HIV-positive KSHV-MCD patients treated with rituximab-based therapy found that the 5-year relapse-free survival was 82% without maintenance rituximab or antiherpes drugs. In addition, all patients with disease relapse were successfully retreated with rituximab-based therapy.[56] Therefore, there is little potential benefit of maintenance therapy because relapse rates are low and remission can be reinduced in a majority of patients. KSHV-MCD patients should be monitored for the development of other Kaposi sarcoma herpesvirus-associated diseases.[43]

Although rituximab has revolutionized KSHV-MCD treatment, there remains a need for rituximab-sparing approaches, especially for patients with concurrent advanced KS, HIV patients with CD4$^+$ counts less than 100 cells/μL, patients allergic to rituximab, and patients in resource-limited settings. Monoclonal antibodies targeting hIL-6 activity have been developed for KSHV-negative (idiopathic) MCD and several rheumatologic conditions and are promising for KSHV-MCD given the role hIL-6 plays in the pathogenesis of symptomatic disease. Siltuximab, a monoclonal antibody that binds directly to hIL-6, is FDA-approved for the treatment of idiopathic MCD but has not been evaluated in KSHV-MCD.[58,59] Tocilizumab, a humanized monoclonal antibody against the IL-6 receptor, is FDA-approved for rheumatoid arthritis and has shown activity in other forms of MCD and also 2 Kaposi sarcoma herpesvirus-associated cases.[60] Targeting hIL-6 is not expected to directly influence vIL-6 activity, which plays an essential role in pathogenesis of symptomatic KSHV-MCD. Therefore, anti-IL6 agents may require combination with other approaches, such as virus-activated cytotoxic therapy.[33] The authors are currently studying tocilizumab in KSHV-MCD in a clinical trial at the NCI (NCT01441063). Pomalidomide has been shown effective against KS, and in the laboratory it can prevent the KSHV-induced down-regulation of MHC-1.[61,62] Based on these findings, the authors' group is exploring the combination of pomalidomide and liposomal doxorubicin in patients with concurrent KS and KSHV-MCD (NCT02659930). The authors hypothesize that combination chemoimmunotherapy will debulk high KS tumor burden while decreasing KSH- driven immune evasion and counteracting paracrine growth signals within the microenvironment.[62]

SUMMARY

KSHV-MCD is a rare and potentially deadly B-cell lymphoproliferative disorder with waxing and waning symptoms that make diagnosis a challenge. Physicians should have a high index of suspicion for KSHV-MCD, especially in high-risk patients. Symptoms and laboratory abnormalities are associated with KSHV lytic activation and elevated inflammatory cytokines. Rituximab-based therapies have led to a drastic improvement, with most recent studies reporting greater than 90% overall 5-year survival.[56] As KSHV-MCD patients continue to live longer with established and experimental treatment approaches, clinicians must remain vigilant for KSHV-MCD relapse and development of other Kaposi sarcoma herpesvirus-associated diseases.

DISCLOSURES

This work was supported by the Intramural Research Program of the National Institutes of Health National Cancer Institute (ZIA BC 011700). Research of the authors is supported in part by a Cooperative Research and Development Agreement between the National Cancer Institute and Celgene. T.S. Uldrick and R. Yarchoan are coinventors on a patent application related to the treatment of Kaposi sarcoma herpesvirus (KSHV)-associated diseases with pomalidomide, and the spouse of R. Yarchoan is a coinventor on a patent related to the measurement of KSHV viral interleukin 6. These inventions were all made as part of their duties as employees of the U.S. Government, and the patents are or will be assigned to U.S. Department of Health and Human Services. The government may convey a portion of the royalties it receives from licensure of its patents to its employee inventors. Finally, R. Yarchoan and T.S. Uldrick have recently conducted clinical research using drugs supplied to the National Cancer Institute by Merck and Co., Hoffman LaRoche, and Bayer Healthcare.

ACKNOWLEDGMENTS

The authors thank Hao-Wei Wang for pathology images.

REFERENCES

1. Oksenhendler E, Duarte M, Soulier J, et al. Multicentric Castleman's disease in HIV infection: a clinical and pathological study of 20 patients. AIDS 1996;10(1): 61–7.
2. Soulier J, Grollet L, Oksenhendler E, et al. Kaposi's sarcoma-associated herpesvirus-like DNA sequences in multicentric Castleman's disease. Blood 1995;86(4): 1276–80.
3. Yoshizaki K, Matsuda T, Nishimoto N, et al. Pathogenic significance of interleukin-6 (IL-6/BSF-2) in Castleman's disease. Blood 1989;74(4):1360–7.
4. Brandt SJ, Bodine DM, Dunbar CE, et al. Dysregulated interleukin 6 expression produces a syndrome resembling Castleman's disease in mice. J Clin Invest 1990;86(2):592–9.
5. Oksenhendler E, Carcelain G, Aoki Y, et al. High levels of human herpesvirus 8 viral load, human interleukin-6, interleukin-10, and C reactive protein correlate with exacerbation of multicentric castleman disease in HIV-infected patients. Blood 2000;96(6):2069–73.
6. Powles T, Stebbing J, Bazeos A, et al. The role of immune suppression and HHV-8 in the increasing incidence of HIV-associated multicentric Castleman's disease. Ann Oncol 2009;20(4):775–9.
7. Bower M, Newsom-Davis T, Naresh K, et al. Clinical features and outcome in HIV-associated multicentric Castleman's disease. J Clin Oncol 2011;29(18):2481–6.
8. Guihot A, Oksenhendler E, Galicier L, et al. Multicentric Castleman disease is associated with polyfunctional effector memory HHV-8-specific CD8+ T cells. Blood 2008;111(3):1387–95.
9. Simard EP, Pfeiffer RM, Engels EA. Cumulative incidence of cancer among individuals with acquired immunodeficiency syndrome in the United States. Cancer 2011;117(5):1089–96.
10. Gao SJ, Kingsley L, Li M, et al. KSHV antibodies among Americans, Italians and Ugandans with and without Kaposi's sarcoma. Nat Med 1996;2(8):925–8.
11. Maskew M, Macphail AP, Whitby D, et al. Prevalence and predictors of kaposi sarcoma herpes virus seropositivity: a cross-sectional analysis of HIV-infected adults initiating ART in Johannesburg, South Africa. Infect Agent Cancer 2011; 6:22.
12. Shebl FM, Dollard SC, Pfeiffer RM, et al. Human herpesvirus 8 seropositivity among sexually active adults in Uganda. PLoS One 2011;6(6):e21286.

13. Gopal S, Liomba NG, Montgomery ND, et al. Characteristics and survival for HIV-associated multicentric Castleman disease in Malawi. J Int AIDS Soc 2015;18: 20122.
14. Uldrick TS, Polizzotto MN, Aleman K, et al. Rituximab plus liposomal doxorubicin in HIV-infected patients with KSHV-associated multicentric Castleman disease. Blood 2014;124(24):3544–52.
15. Gopal S, Wood WA, Lee SJ, et al. Meeting the challenge of hematologic malignancies in sub-Saharan Africa. Blood 2012;119(22):5078–87.
16. Polizzotto MN, Uldrick TS, Wyvill KM, et al. Clinical features and outcomes of patients with symptomatic Kaposi sarcoma Herpesvirus (KSHV)-associated inflammation: prospective characterization of KSHV inflammatory cytokine syndrome (KICS). Clin Infect Dis 2016;62(6):730–8.
17. Uldrick TS, Wang V, O'Mahony D, et al. An interleukin-6-related systemic inflammatory syndrome in patients co-infected with Kaposi sarcoma-associated herpesvirus and HIV but without Multicentric Castleman disease. Clin Infect Dis 2010;51(3):350–8.
18. Coscoy L, Ganem D. Kaposi's sarcoma-associated herpesvirus encodes two proteins that block cell surface display of MHC class I chains by enhancing their endocytosis. Proc Natl Acad Sci U S A 2000;97(14):8051–6.
19. Sanchez DJ, Gumperz JE, Ganem D. Regulation of CD1d expression and function by a herpesvirus infection. J Clin Invest 2005;115(5):1369–78.
20. Sbihi Z, Dossier A, Boutboul D, et al. iNKT and memory B-cell alterations in HHV-8 multicentric Castleman disease. Blood 2017;129(7):855–65.
21. Chung BK, Tsai K, Allan LL, et al. Innate immune control of EBV-infected B cells by invariant natural killer T cells. Blood 2013;122(15):2600–8.
22. Hassman LM, Ellison TJ, Kedes DH. KSHV infects a subset of human tonsillar B cells, driving proliferation and plasmablast differentiation. J Clin Invest 2011; 121(2):752–68.
23. Parravicini C, Chandran B, Corbellino M, et al. Differential viral protein expression in Kaposi's sarcoma-associated herpesvirus-infected diseases: Kaposi's sarcoma, primary effusion lymphoma, and multicentric Castleman's disease. Am J Pathol 2000;156(3):743–9.
24. Staskus KA, Sun R, Miller G, et al. Cellular tropism and viral interleukin-6 expression distinguish human herpesvirus 8 involvement in Kaposi's sarcoma, primary effusion lymphoma, and multicentric Castleman's disease. J Virol 1999;73(5): 4181–7.
25. Katano H, Sato Y, Kurata T, et al. Expression and localization of human herpesvirus 8-encoded proteins in primary effusion lymphoma, Kaposi's sarcoma, and multicentric Castleman's disease. Virology 2000;269(2):335–44.
26. Polizzotto MN, Uldrick TS, Wang V, et al. Human and viral interleukin-6 and other cytokines in Kaposi sarcoma herpesvirus-associated multicentric Castleman disease. Blood 2013;122(26):4189–98.
27. Bower M, Veraitch O, Szydlo R, et al. Cytokine changes during rituximab therapy in HIV-associated multicentric Castleman disease. Blood 2009;113(19):4521–4.
28. Osborne J, Moore PS, Chang Y. KSHV-encoded viral IL-6 activates multiple human IL-6 signaling pathways. Hum Immunol 1999;60(10):921–7.
29. Moore PS, Boshoff C, Weiss RA, et al. Molecular mimicry of human cytokine and cytokine response pathway genes by KSHV. Science 1996;274(5293):1739–44.
30. Aoki Y, Jones KD, Tosato G. Kaposi's sarcoma-associated herpesvirus-encoded interleukin-6. J Hematother Stem Cell Res 2000;9(2):137–45.

31. Aoki Y, Tosato G, Fonville TW, et al. Serum viral interleukin-6 in AIDS-related multi-centric Castleman disease. Blood 2001;97(8):2526–7.
32. Hu D, Wang V, Yang M, et al. Induction of Kaposi's Sarcoma-associated Herpes-virus-encoded viral interleukin-6 by X-box binding protein 1. J Virol 2015;90(1): 368–78.
33. Suthaus J, Stuhlmann-Laeisz C, Tompkins VS, et al. HHV-8-encoded viral IL-6 col-laborates with mouse IL-6 in the development of multicentric Castleman disease in mice. Blood 2012;119(22):5173–81.
34. Ballon G, Akar G, Cesarman E. Systemic expression of Kaposi sarcoma herpes-virus (KSHV) Vflip in endothelial cells leads to a profound proinflammatory pheno-type and myeloid lineage remodeling in vivo. PLoS Pathog 2015;11(1):e1004581.
35. Polizzotto MN, Millo C, Uldrick TS, et al. 18F-fluorodeoxyglucose positron emis-sion tomography in Kaposi Sarcoma Herpesvirus-associated multicentric Castle-man Disease: correlation with activity, severity, inflammatory and virologic parameters. J Infect Dis 2015;212(8):1250–60.
36. Newsom-Davis T, Bower M, Wildfire A, et al. Resolution of AIDS-related Castle-man's disease with anti-CD20 monoclonal antibodies is associated with declining IL-6 and TNF-alpha levels. Leuk Lymphoma 2004;45(9):1939–41.
37. Fardet L, Blum L, Kerob D, et al. Human herpesvirus 8-associated hemophago-cytic lymphohistiocytosis in human immunodeficiency virus-infected patients. Clin Infect Dis 2003;37(2):285–91.
38. Dupin N, Diss TL, Kellam P, et al. HHV-8 is associated with a plasmablastic variant of Castleman disease that is linked to HHV-8-positive plasmablastic lym-phoma. Blood 2000;95(4):1406–12.
39. Chadburn A, Hyjek EM, Tam W, et al. Immunophenotypic analysis of the Kaposi sarcoma herpesvirus (KSHV; HHV-8)-infected B cells in HIV+ multicentric Castle-man disease (MCD). Histopathology 2008;53(5):513–24.
40. Du MQ, Diss TC, Liu H, et al. KSHV- and EBV-associated germinotropic lympho-proliferative disorder. Blood 2002;100(9):3415–8.
41. Wang HW, Pittaluga S, Jaffe ES. Multicentric Castleman disease: where are we now? Semin Diagn Pathol 2016;33(5):294–306.
42. Venkataraman G, Uldrick TS, Aleman K, et al. Bone marrow findings in HIV-positive patients with Kaposi sarcoma herpesvirus-associated multicentric Cas-tleman disease. Am J Clin Pathol 2013;139(5):651–61.
43. Oksenhendler E, Boulanger E, Galicier L, et al. High incidence of Kaposi sarcoma-associated herpesvirus-related non-Hodgkin lymphoma in patients with HIV infection and multicentric Castleman disease. Blood 2002;99(7):2331–6.
44. Gerard L, Michot JM, Burcheri S, et al. Rituximab decreases the risk of lymphoma in patients with HIV-associated multicentric Castleman disease. Blood 2012; 119(10):2228–33.
45. Bower M. How I treat HIV-associated multicentric Castleman disease. Blood 2010;116(22):4415–21.
46. Aaron L, Lidove O, Yousry C, et al. Human herpesvirus 8-positive Castleman dis-ease in human immunodeficiency virus-infected patients: the impact of highly active antiretroviral therapy. Clin Infect Dis 2002;35(7):880–2.
47. Samji H, Cescon A, Hogg RS, et al. Closing the gap: increases in life expectancy among treated HIV-positive individuals in the United States and Canada. PLoS One 2013;8(12):e81355.
48. Bower M, Powles T, Williams S, et al. Brief communication: rituximab in HIV-associated multicentric Castleman disease. Ann Intern Med 2007;147(12):836–9.

49. Gerard L, Berezne A, Galicier L, et al. Prospective study of rituximab in chemotherapy-dependent human immunodeficiency virus associated multicentric Castleman's disease: ANRS 117 CastlemaB Trial. J Clin Oncol 2007;25(22): 3350–6.
50. Dossier A, Meignin V, Fieschi C, et al. Human herpesvirus 8-related Castleman disease in the absence of HIV infection. Clin Infect Dis 2013;56(6):833–42.
51. Casper C, Nichols WG, Huang ML, et al. Remission of HHV-8 and HIV-associated multicentric Castleman disease with ganciclovir treatment. Blood 2004;103(5): 1632–4.
52. Davis DA, Singer KE, Reynolds IP, et al. Hypoxia enhances the phosphorylation and cytotoxicity of ganciclovir and zidovudine in Kaposi's sarcoma-associated herpesvirus infected cells. Cancer Res 2007;67(14):7003–10.
53. Uldrick TS, Polizzotto MN, Aleman K, et al. High-dose zidovudine plus valganciclovir for Kaposi sarcoma herpesvirus-associated multicentric Castleman disease: a pilot study of virus-activated cytotoxic therapy. Blood 2011;117(26): 6977–86.
54. Neuville S, Agbalika F, Rabian C, et al. Failure of rituximab in human immunodeficiency virus-associated multicentric Castleman disease. Am J Hematol 2005; 79(4):337–9.
55. Buchler T, Dubash S, Lee V, et al. Rituximab failure in fulminant multicentric HIV/human herpesvirus 8-associated Castleman's disease with multiorgan failure: report of two cases. AIDS 2008;22(13):1685–7.
56. Pria AD, Pinato D, Roe J, et al. Relapse of HHV8-positive multicentric Castleman disease following rituximab-based therapy in HIV-positive patients. Blood 2017; 129(15):2143–7.
57. Stebbing J, Adams C, Sanitt A, et al. Plasma HHV8 DNA predicts relapse in individuals with HIV-associated multicentric Castleman disease. Blood 2011; 118(2):271–5.
58. Trikha M, Corringham R, Klein B, et al. Targeted anti-interleukin-6 monoclonal antibody therapy for cancer: a review of the rationale and clinical evidence. Clin Cancer Res 2003;9(13):4653–65.
59. van Rhee F, Wong RS, Munshi N, et al. Siltuximab for multicentric Castleman's disease: a randomised, double-blind, placebo-controlled trial. Lancet Oncol 2014;15(9):966–74.
60. Nishimoto N, Kanakura Y, Aozasa K, et al. Humanized anti-interleukin-6 receptor antibody treatment of multicentric Castleman disease. Blood 2005;106(8): 2627–32.
61. Polizzotto MN, Uldrick TS, Wyvill KM, et al. Pomalidomide for symptomatic Kaposi's Sarcoma in people with and without HIV infection: a phase I/II study. J Clin Oncol 2016;34(34):4125–31.
62. Davis DA, Mishra S, Anagho HA, et al. Restoration of immune surface molecules in Kaposi sarcoma-associated herpes virus infected cells by lenalidomide and pomalidomide. Oncotarget 2017;8(31):50342–58.

Treatment of Idiopathic Castleman Disease

Frits van Rhee, MD, PhD, MRCP(UK), FRCPath*, Amy Greenway, BS, CRS, Katie Stone, BS, CRS

KEYWORDS

- Castleman disease • Treatment • Rituximab • Corticosteroids • Chemotherapy
- Tocilizumab • Siltuximab

KEY POINTS

- Accurate diagnosis of the different varieties of multicentric Castleman disease is critical to guiding therapy.
- Monoclonal antibodies targeting the interleukin-6 signaling pathway are the best-studied agents in idiopathic multicentric Castleman disease and are front-line therapy for more severely ill patients.
- Rituximab has not been systematically studied, but is commonly used as initial therapy for more indolent idiopathic multicentric Castleman disease.
- Chemotherapy and immunomodulatory drugs are best reserved for the relapse setting.
- Autologous stem cell transplantation should be considered for patients with coexistent POEMS syndrome.

INTRODUCTION

Castleman disease (CD) is a rare, heterogeneous lymphoproliferative disorder first defined in 1954.[1] The variable manifestations of CD and infrequent presentation outside of academic centers of excellence result in difficulty of diagnosis and management of the disease. CD may be divided into 2 major forms. Unicentric CD (UCD) is typically a slow-growing solitary mass occurring at a single anatomic site; although the enlarging mass may compress vital structures, surgical excision is generally curative. In contrast, multicentric CD (MCD) affects multiple lymph node stations and often presents with lymphadenopathy, fever, weight loss, fatigue, edema, anemia, and hypoalbuminemia.[2–4] In severe cases, patients may develop hepatosplenomegaly, massive ascites, pleural effusions, or organ failure, and both UCD and MCD

Disclosure Statement: F. van Rhee has received research funding from Janssen Pharmaceuticals.
UAMS Myeloma Institute, University of Arkansas for Medical Sciences, 4301 West Markham, #816, Little Rock, AR 72205, USA
* Corresponding author.
E-mail address: vanrheefrits@uams.edu

Hematol Oncol Clin N Am 32 (2018) 89–106
https://doi.org/10.1016/j.hoc.2017.09.008   **hemonc.theclinics.com**

sometimes progress to non-Hodgkin lymphoma (NHL). MCD often concomitantly presents in the context of infection with the human immunodeficiency virus (HIV) and/or human herpesvirus 8 (HHV8). However, approximately 50% of patients with MCD who are negative for HIV and HHV8 comprise a subgroup that has recently been termed as idiopathic MCD (iMCD), as no causative etiology has been established. The rarity of CD has unfortunately limited the ability to perform systematic studies providing solid evidence of superiority of therapeutic strategies. In this article, we report on evidence for various treatments to synthesize a treatment algorithm for the practicing physician.

CLINICAL SYMPTOMATOLOGY OF MULTICENTRIC CASTLEMAN DISEASE AND ROLE OF INTERLEUKIN-6

Interleukin-6 (IL6) is a pleiotropic cytokine that plays a pivotal role in the pathogenesis and clinical symptomatology in many patients with iMCD. The notion that IL6 plays a causative role in iMCD is supported by several clinical and experimental observations. Clinically, MCD is characterized by a proinflammatory syndrome giving rise to the so-called B-symptoms comprising fevers, night sweats, malaise, and weight loss.[5] The C-reactive protein (CRP) is commonly elevated and is considered to be a surrogate marker for IL6 bioactivity.[6] Elevated fibrinogen levels in the setting of a systemic inflammatory response can cause deep venous thrombosis and other thrombo-embolic disorders. IL6 is an important growth, differentiation, and survival factor for both plasma cells and lymphocytes contributing to lymph node enlargement, plasmacytic infiltration, hepatosplenomegaly, and reactive bone marrow plasmacytosis with polyclonal hypergammaglobulenemia. IL6 also dysregulates the humoral immune response resulting in positive antinuclear antibody assays in approximately one-third of the patients, immune thrombocytopenia, hemolytic anemia, as well as a host of other autoimmune phenomena likely caused by expansion of $CD5^+$ B-lymphocytes.[7,8] Together with other cytokines, IL6 also induces polyclonal T-cell outgrowth reflected by the presence of activated $CD8^+$ T cells and increased soluble IL2 receptor levels. During the inflammatory response, IL6 increases the production of the peptide hormone regulator of iron homeostasis, hepcidin, by the liver. Hepcidin reduces intestinal iron absorption and impairs release of stored iron from macrophages, thus causing anemia.[9,10] Furthermore, IL6 inhibits albumin production by the liver, leading to hypoalbuminemia. IL6-induced vascular endothelial growth factor (VEGF) secretion promotes angiogenesis and vascular permeability; the latter combines with hypoalbuminemia to induce edema, ascites, pleural and pericardial effusions, and generalized anasarca due to vascular leak syndrome. In severe cases of iMCD, renal failure occurs, often due to thrombotic microangiopathy and multiorgan failure can ensue, resulting in death.

The role of IL6 is further underscored by the observation that surgical debulking with removal of lymph nodes can lead to rapid reductions in IL6 levels and clinical improvement.[11] Patients who have other malignancies that overproduce IL6 can have pathologic changes in enlarged lymph nodes that resemble CD and that resolve following surgical resection or with monoclonal antibody (mAb)-mediated IL6 blockade.[12,13] IL6 levels can also wax and wane in step with the severity of clinical symptoms.[5] Mice in which IL6 is overexpressed using retroviral transduced bone marrow cells develop a Castleman-like syndrome.[14,15] In IL6 transgenic mice, a similar MCD picture emerges, which is ameliorated by neutralization of IL6 with an antibody directed at the IL6 receptor (IL6R).[16,17] IL6 transcription is regulated by the transcription factor C/EBPβ and CCAAT/enhancer binding protein-β knockout transgenic mice develop lymphadenopathy, splenomegaly, and other Castleman features.[18] Interestingly viral IL6 expression in mice also yields an MCD-like phenotype. However, this phenotype is mitigated when the viral IL6 transgene is expressed into IL6 knockout mice suggesting that even in virally induced MCD, endogenous IL6 remains a critical cofactor.[19] Recombinant IL6 given to humans also leads to a syndrome resembling MCD.[20] Polymorphism of a minor *IL6R* allele is more prevalent in iMCD and may result in increased IL6 *trans*-signaling.[5] The exact nature of the IL6 secreting cell(s) has not been elucidated and proposed candidates include B-lymphocytes, plasma cells, monocytes, macrophages, follicular dendritic cells, and stromal cells.[11,21–24] Although, IL6 may not be of pathogenic significance in all patients, the aforementioned findings have sparked the interest in mAbs therapeutically targeting the IL6 signaling cascade as described later in this article.

Multicentric Castleman Disease Classification and Therapy

It is important to render a correct diagnosis and recognize the distinct variants of MCD, which require different therapy. Until recently, most of the medical literature has focused on patients with HIV who develop MCD and are coinfected with HHV8. HHV8-accociated MCD is a separate entity requiring a different therapeutic approach usually based on rituximab with or without etoposide or doxorubicin. HIV-induced immunosuppression can lead to lytic replication of immunoglobulin (Ig)M/λ restricted plasmablasts, which often express CD20, in the lymph node mantle zones and interfollicular areas that can be efficiently targeted with rituximab.[25–28] HHV8 encodes for the viral orthologue of IL6, which can induce the release of human IL6 and precipitate a cytokine storm responsible for the clinical symptomatology. Although HHV8 reactivation is classically associated with HIV infection, cases of HHV8-positive MCD have also been reported without concomitant HIV infection. Furthermore, these HIV-negative cases have similar clinical presentation compared with their HIV-positive counterparts, justifying their classification as a single clinicopathological entity, which require a similar therapeutic approach.[29–32] HHV8-associated MCD can be recognized by either a positive HHV8 latency associated nuclear antigen test of lymph node tissue or the detection of circulating HHV8 DNA in the peripheral blood indicative of actively replicating HHV8. HHV8 serology should not be used to identify HHV8-positive MCD because it has poor sensitivity and specificity.[29]

It has become increasingly clear that there is a significant population of patients with MCD who are not infected with HIV or HHV8 and are referred to as iMCD. Until recently, there were no uniform diagnostic criteria for iMCD. An international working group from 8 countries has now defined consensus criteria for the diagnosis of iMCD. Patients should have enlargement of 2 or more lymph node stations and lymph node pathology compatible with iMCD. Other diseases that can give rise to similar pathology should be actively excluded. These include autoimmune disorders, such as systemic lupus erythematosus, infections, or lymphoma. Further, patients should have at least 2 of 11 minor criteria, of which one should be a laboratory parameter reflecting an active inflammatory state.[33] The establishment of these diagnostic criteria will help to evaluate patients, assist physicians to arrive at the correct diagnosis, and lead to the implementation of appropriate therapy as discussed later in this article.

A subgroup of patients labeled as having TAFRO syndrome (*T*hrombocytopenia, *A*nasarca, *F*ever, *R*eticulin Fibrosis, and *O*rganomegaly) appear to be more severely ill and often have renal impairment and have worse outcome than other patients with iMCD.[34–40] The clinical course of TAFRO syndrome is more aggressive and characterized by frequent steroid refractoriness requiring additional therapies, including tocilizumab, cytoxic agents, cyclosporin, and rituximab, as reported by Iwaki and colleagues[39] in a series of 25 patients. Three of 7 patients did not respond to anti-IL6 mAb therapy. Further, patients often have normal gamma globulin levels, elevated alkaline phosphatase, and relatively modest size lymphadenopathy. Future studies will have to determine whether TAFRO is a distinct clinical entity in the iMCD spectrum with its own pathophysiology and unique cytokine profile, because IL6 seems to be less elevated than in non-TAFRO patients with plasmacytic variant of iMCD. It may be even be that some of these patients will require novel therapeutic approaches.

It is important to realize that the distinction between UCD and iMCD is not always absolute and that there are patients who have more limited lymph node involvement and are referred to as having "regional" or "oligocentric" CD. Often these patients have no associated B-symptomatology or proinflammatory markers, and these patients should be managed more like UCD. A further group of patients requiring different treatment are patients suffering from both POEMS (polyneuropathy, organomegaly, endocrinopathy, monoclonal gammopathy, skin changes) and MCD, or those who have MCD with features of POEMS, but not meeting formal diagnostic criteria of POEMS.[33,41]

Therapeutic Options for Idiopathic Multicentric Castleman Disease

Overview

A large variety of different treatments have been used to manage iMCD. These therapeutic modalities include surgery, corticosteroids, rituximab, combination chemotherapy, autologous stem cell transplantation (ASCT), mAbs interrupting the IL6 signaling cascade, novel agents such as bortezomib, thalidomide, the IL1-antagonist, anakinra, and other immunomodulatory molecules, such as interferon-α and all-trans retinoic acid. Most of these reports are based on small series, case reports, literature reviews, and retrospective analyses of institutional experiences. Only one prospective randomized placebo-controlled trial has been conducted in iMCD studying the efficacy of the IL6-neutralizing mAb siltuximab.[42] Interpretation of the data is further hampered by the previous lack of uniform diagnostic criteria, clinical heterogeneity of the various patient populations, likely bias toward reporting positive findings, important missing clinical parameters (eg, HHV8 status), and inconsistency in measuring outcome parameters. There are also presently no biomarkers that predict response to a specific therapy. Treatment recommendations are therefore not based on hard clinical evidence, but rather on the expert opinion of those actively involved in the care of patients with iMCD and with knowledge of the literature.

Overall outcome of idiopathic multicentric Castleman disease

Several studies have reported on the outcome of MCD. Dispenzieri and colleagues[43] reported on a retrospective series of 113 patients treated at the Mayo Clinic and the University of Nebraska. The 5-year overall survival (OS) was only 65% for patients with MCD versus 91% for patients with UCD. With a median follow-up of 5.8 years, 37 patients had died. This patient cohort was not formally tested for HIV or HHV8, but none had clinical AIDS at diagnosis nor subsequently during follow-up. Because of existing referral patterns, this patient population was enriched for POEMS syndrome, which likely impacted outcome. The 5-year OS for patients without coexistent POEMS syndrome was respectively 65% for patients without peripheral neuropathy and only 51% for patients who did suffer from peripheral neuropathy. The most indolent course was observed in patients who had POEMS syndrome with coexistent osteosclerotic lesions who enjoyed a 5-year OS of 90%, contrasting to those without osteosclerosis who fared worse with a dismal 5-year OS of 27%. Most of these patients were treated with steroids or chemotherapy. One can only speculate that patients with MCD without POEMS may have benefited from modern treatment approaches with rituximab or anti-IL6 agents, whereas those with POEMS would presently be considered for ASCT. Talat and Schulte[44] reported on 384 HIV-negative patients with MCD, of whom 148 had 3-year disease-free survival (DFS) data. Patients with plasmacytic variant of MCD had a 3-year DFS of only 45%. Three-year DFS was significantly better in younger patients (<37), female patients, or those with hyaline-vascular versus plasmacytic pathology. It was not possible to evaluate how outcome was influenced by different therapeutic interventions because treatment details were not supplied. Liu and colleagues[45] performed a systematic literature review of 114 patients with iMCD who were treated with a variety of modalities, including steroids, chemotherapy, rituximab, and anti-IL6 mAbs. The 2-year OS was 88% with a follow-up of 29 months; 27 (22%) patients died during the follow-up period. Interestingly, 24 patients had a separate malignant disease (solid tumor, n = 13; hematologic malignancy, n = 11) either at diagnosis of iMCD or during follow-up. Two-year survival was significantly better in patients without a malignancy (92% vs 70%). Other adverse prognostic features included age older than 37 years, plasmacytic histology, thrombocytopenia, hypergammaglobulinemia, and features of TAFRO syndrome, although statistical significance was achieved only for a concomitant malignancy. Taken together, these studies did not identify any consistent prognostic factors across all studies, but findings do poignantly highlight that iMCD is a life-threatening disorder for many patients, with DFS and OS rates that are typically seen with malignant disorders.

Surgery and irradiation

Complete surgical resection is rarely feasible in iMCD, although it is often curative for UCD. In a series of 127 patients with MCD, debulking surgery did not improve 10-year OS whether surgery was performed alone or as adjunct therapy.[46] Other investigators have also not reported meaningful contributions of surgery in the MCD setting.[47,48] There is no role for splenectomy as a diagnostic procedure, but it can occasionally be useful in the management of therapy-resistant hemolytic anemia.[49] Similarly, there is no established role for radiotherapy in MCD.[50] Patients with coexistent POEMS syndrome and a localized plasmacytoma may benefit from local radiotherapy, although it is not clear to what extent any associated iMCD would be improved.

Corticosteroids

Corticosteroids can suppress the hypercytokinemia in iMCD, but this typically requires high-dose therapy, which cannot be sustained for a prolonged period. Long-term disease control and lasting remissions with steroid therapy are uncommon, and relapses occur frequently on cessation of therapy or during steroid tapering.[47,48,50–53] Prolonged steroid therapy also increases the risk of bacterial infection and sepsis. Steroids can be useful in achieving initial disease control in combination with chemotherapy, rituximab, or anti-IL6 mAb therapy and should be seen as an adjunct therapy. Selected patients may benefit from low-dose steroid therapy in the maintenance setting, usually in combination with other agents.[54,55]

Chemotherapy

There has been no systematic evaluation of chemotherapy in controlled studies. Typically, chemotherapy regimens have been adopted from NHL therapy and include CHOP (cyclophosphamide, doxorubicin, vincristine [Oncovin], prednisolone) or CVAD (cyclophosphamide, vincristine, adriamycin, etoposide)-like regimens with or without rituximab. The authors of this article have used combination chemotherapy used for myeloma, for example, VDTPACE (velcade [bortezomib], dexamethasone, thalidomide, cisplatinum, adriamycin, cyclophosphamide, etoposide).[56] Lasting remissions have been reported by some investigators. In one early report, 27% of patients had a sustained remission,[47] whereas Chronowski and colleagues[50] observed a progression-free survival (PFS) varying from 23 to 119 months in 4 of 9 responding patients. Zhu and colleagues[57] reported on 10 patients with iMCD treated with CHOP or COP (cyclophosphamide, vincristine [Oncovin], prednisolone). One achieved complete response (CR), and 6 had a partial response (PR), with all 7 patients remaining alive with a median follow-up of 34 months. However, others failed to document meaningful responses.[52,53] In a recent retrospective literature review, cytotoxic therapy induced CR in 19 of 43 patients with a median time to treatment failure of 6 months.[45] It seems appropriate to reserve chemotherapy for the salvage setting in view of its toxicity and the availability of other active agents, such as rituximab and the anti-IL6 mAbs, tocilizumab and siltuximab. A notable exception to this recommendation may be critically ill patients who fail to respond to mAb therapy and steroids. In this setting, prompt institution of combination chemotherapy can be literally lifesaving.

Rituximab

The introduction of rituximab in patients with HIV-positive, HHV8-positive MCD has greatly improved outcome in several studies and significantly decreased the risk of transformation to lymphoma.[27,28,58–60] Rituximab eliminates a reservoir of CD20+ B-cells and plasmablasts in which HHV8 lytically replicates explaining its activity in HHV8-positive MCD. Rituximab has also been widely used for the treatment of iMCD and is recommended by the National Comprehensive Cancer Network guidelines as one of the primary therapies for iMCD (www.nccn.org). However, there have been no clinical trials assessing the efficacy of rituximab and there have been remarkably few case reports or series in the literature pertaining to iMCD.[61–63] In one report describing 25 cases of iMCD, the CR and PR rates with rituximab as first-line therapy were 20% and 48%, respectively, with the anti-IL6 mAb siltuximab outperforming rituximab in terms of PFS.[40] More encouragingly, in another series, 5 of 8 patients achieved CR with rituximab as sole therapy and only one failed therapy.[45] Despite the lack of robust data, the use of rituximab is firmly entrenched in the treatment of iMCD and perceived as a therapy of limited duration, which can induce durable remissions. Furthermore, many oncologists feel very comfortable with rituximab, which was first approved in 1997 and is widely used for the treatment of a variety of B-lymphoid malignancies, including follicular and diffuse large-cell lymphoma, chronic lymphocytic leukemia, and Waldenström macroglobulinemia. Although no formal clinical studies are anticipated in the future, the ACCELERATE registry of the Castleman Disease Collaborative Network (CDCN) will play an important future role in collecting "real-life" data regarding the efficacy of rituximab and help to further clarify the role of rituximab in iMCD (www.cdcn.org).

Anti-IL6 agents

IL6 binds to the IL6R, which is present as soluble or membrane-bound, producing a complex that binds to the glycoprotein 130 (gp130), resulting in dimerization and activating of the Janus kinase/signal transducers and activators of transcription (JAK/STAT) signaling cascade promoting cell survival and proliferation. The introduction of mAbs directed at the IL6 pathway is an important contribution to the therapeutic armamentarium for iMCD. Two mAbs that target the IL6 signaling cascade have been extensively studied in iMCD (**Fig. 1**). Tocilizumab is a humanized Igκ mAb that binds to both the soluble and membrane-bound forms of the IL6R. Siltuximab is a chimeric human-murine Igκ mAb, which directly binds to IL6. The first clinical application of an IL6 mAb in a patient with CD was reported by Beck and colleagues[64] using the murine antibody BE-8. Although the antibody induced a clinical response, symptoms rapidly recurred after cessation of therapy. The antibody had a short half-life and was unable to block large quantities of IL6, leading to the search for more potent antibodies.

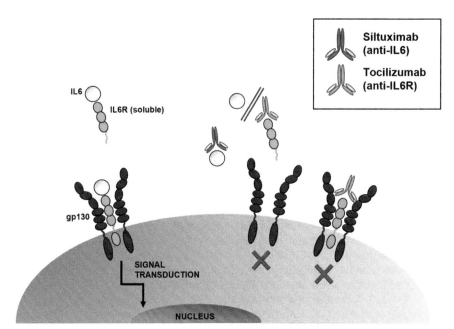

Fig. 1. Blockade of IL6 signaling by monoclonal antibodies. IL6 signaling occurs when IL6 interacts with either the soluble or membrane-bound form of IL6R. In association with the signal transducer gp130, this complex results in dimerization and activation of the JAK/STAT signaling cascade. The mAbs siltuximab and tocilizumab disrupt IL6 signaling by blocking IL6 or the IL6R (in soluble or membrane-bound form), respectively.

Sato and colleagues[65] subsequently created a humanized anti-IL6R antibody by grafting the complementarity region of the murine anti-IL6R antibody, PM-1, onto human IgG creating rhPM-1, later referred to as MRA or tocilizumab. Nishimoto and colleagues[66] first reported on the treatment of 7 patients with MCD in Japan with tocilizumab. All 7 patients tested negative for HIV and HHV8. Tocilizumab improved clinical symptoms and reduced levels of CRP, fibrinogen, serum amyloid A, and gamma globulins in all patients. There was also virtual complete resolution of lymph adenopathy demonstrated by computed tomography (CT) scanning, and repeat lymph node biopsy during therapy showed improvement in histologic changes with reduction in number and size of follicles as well as decrease in vascularity in terms of hyaline capillaries in the interfollicular areas. In a subsequent open-label multicenter, prospective study 28 patients with iMCD, all with plasmacytic variant, were treated with tocilizumab (8 mg/kg) every 2 weeks for 16 weeks followed by continued dosing at the discretion of the investigator, mostly at 2-weekly intervals (53% of patients) or 4-weekly intervals (18%). Two patients were seropositive for HHV8 and all were HIV-negative. All patients were significantly symptomatic, had elevated CRP and IL6 levels, and most had severe anemia and hypoalbuminemia.

Patients showed significant reduction in lymphadenopathy by 16 weeks, with 52% of patients achieving lymph node sizes of less than 1 cm by 1 year. Apart from resolution of symptoms such as fatigue, nutritional status, cholesterol, and body mass improved in all patients. There was rapid normalization in several key indicators of systemic inflammation, such as CRP, albumin, and IgG. Eight of 12 patients with iMCD-related skin disorders experienced improvement. Fifteen patients were on steroid therapy at the onset of tocilizumab therapy and 11 of these were able to discontinue steroids or decrease the dose. At the time of reporting, all but 1 patient continued to receive MRA therapy for more than 3 years and treatment was well tolerated with only 2 patients experiencing a serious adverse event, cellulitis, possibly related to tocilizumab. Fourteen patients had mild and transient infusion reactions. Overall, both studies showed that tocilizumab had significant activity in the treatment of iMCD with acceptable toxicity. As a result of these initial 2 studies, tocilizumab was registered as an orphan drug for MCD in 2005 in Japan, becoming the first approved drug for the therapy of MCD anywhere in the world.

In a follow-up report in 2007, by which time 35 patients had been treated, 30 (86%) remained on study over a period of 5 years with continued response. Furthermore, pulmonary diffuse hyperplasia, which is much more common in the Asian population, was present in 31 patients and showed significant improvement.[67] The safety and efficacy of tocilizumab has been confirmed over the years in numerous case reports and small series.[68–70] Tocilizumab has also been used successfully in the pediatric population.[71] The most common side effects are increases in bilirubin, hypercholesterolemia, and mild thrombocytopenia.[72]

Siltuximab is an IL6 neutralizing mAb, which prevents IL6 from binding to both the soluble and membrane-bound IL6R. It has a high affinity for human IL6, but does not bind to viral IL6. A prospective open-label study with 7 cohorts enrolled 67 patients, including 37 with iMCD, 17 with NHL, and 13 with multiple myeloma.[73,74] The first 5 cohorts studied escalating siltuximab doses: 3 mg/kg every 2 weeks, 6 mg/kg every 2 weeks, 12 mg/kg every 3 weeks, 6 mg/kg weekly, and 12 mg/kg every 2 weeks. Cohort 6 evaluated 12 mg/kg given at a shorter infusion time (1 hour rather than 2 hours). Cohort 7 was an expansion cohort confined to patients with iMCD who received siltuximab at 9 or 12 mg/kg via a 1-hour infusion. The overall response rate in iMCD in terms of reduction of lymphadenopathy was 52% (CR, n = 1; PR, n = 11). Three patients had an unconfirmed PR, 20 stable disease, and only 1 had disease progression.

There was a relation between siltuximab dose and response, with 73% of patients receiving 12 mg/kg responding versus 33% given lower doses. The CR and 8 of the 11 PRs were seen at the dose level of 12 mg/kg. Responses were seen in all histopathologic subtypes: hyaline-vascular (5 of 18), mixed-cellularity (1 of 2), and plasmacytic (6 of 12). The median time to progression was not reached with a follow-up of 29 months. A so-called Clinical Benefit Response (improvement in hemoglobin, weight, decrease in anorexia, fever/night sweats, and lymphadenopathy) was observed in 87% of patients, with 43% improving in ≥ 4 parameters. The most frequent side effects were thrombocytopenia, hypertriglyceridemia, and neutropenia. The incidence of serious infection across the Phase I and extensions study was 0.02 per patient year. No opportunistic infections were seen, although approximately a quarter to a third of patients did receive herpes zoster prophylaxis. Nineteen patients with iMCD went on to receive treatment in an extension study for a median of 5.1 years (range 3.4–7.2) and no disease relapse or cumulative toxicity was observed.[42] Eight of the 19 patients were able to reduce the dose interval to 6-weekly infusions.

In a subsequent randomized, double-blind, placebo-controlled Phase II study conducted in 19 countries, 79 patients were assigned to either siltuximab 11 mg/kg every 3 weeks (n = 53) or best supportive care (n = 26), allowing for prednisone 1 mg/kg (or equivalent).[55] The primary endpoint was durable tumor and symptomatic response defined as PR or CR by modified Cheson criteria and ≥ 18 weeks' improvement or stabilization of 34 MCD-related symptoms. A significantly higher tumor and symptomatic response was seen in patients treated with siltuximab (34% vs 0%), with 17 patients reaching a PR and 1 a CR. The median time to a symptomatic response was 33 days. However, involution of lymphadenopathy with siltuximab was more gradual, with a median time to response of 155 days. Median time to treatment failure was not reached in the siltuximab arm versus 134 days in the placebo arm. Median time to next treatment was not reached with siltuximab and 280 days with placebo. Fifty-nine percent of patients on the siltuximab arm remained on therapy, compared with 19% in the placebo arm. The tumor response rate (38% vs 4%), durable symptomatic response (57% vs 19%), and complete resolution of symptoms (25% vs 0%) were all superior in the siltuximab arm. There were rapid reductions in CRP, hepcidin, ferritin, fibrinogen, and increases in hemoglobin and albumin.[55,75] Patients reported improvements in iMCD symptoms, such as fatigue and weakness, and objectively reversal of muscle wasting was noted by CT-scanning.[76,77] The adverse event profile was similar to that observed in the Phase I study. Subgroup analyses showed that all durable tumor and symptomatic responses occurred in patients with plasmacytic or mixed-cellularity pathology. In patients with hyaline-vascular pathology, benefit in tumor and symptomatic response were observed as assessed by the investigators rather than central review. Also, the median time to treatment failure in this subgroup was longer with siltuximab compared with placebo (206 vs 70 days). As previously discussed in the Phase I study, clinical responses were observed in patients with hyaline-vascular pathology suggesting that this group of patients with iMCD may still derive benefit from siltuximab therapy. Based on these data, siltuximab was approved for iMCD in the United States, Europe, and Canada in 2014 and in Brazil in 2015.

In clinical practice, both tocilizumab and siltuximab appear equally effective in the management of iMCD and have a similar toxicity profile. Mild thrombocytopenia is common, as are increases in cholesterol. Occasional mild elevation of bilirubin levels occurs. Disadvantages of both drugs are that treatment is not curative and is essentially life-long because relapses have been reported on discontinuation of therapy. However, in many patients, the dosing intervals can be extended. Future studies will have to answer the question, whether some patients remain in remission off therapy and can be managed with a more limited treatment course.

Immunomodulatory agents

A variety of other agents have been reported to have activity in iMCD, mostly in case reports. IL1 is upstream of IL6 in the inflammatory pathway and activates nuclear factor kappa B (NF-κB), leading to transcription of proinflammatory cytokines, including IL6. There have been reports of patients responding to the IL1β receptor antagonist, anakinra. One patient had failed tocilizumab, whereas the response in the second patient was partial and this patient later received tocilizumab.[78,79] Bortezomib similarly inhibits the NF-κB pathway and has been used alone or in combination with other drugs to treat several patients.[80–82] Thalidomide is a potent immunomodulatory agent, which inhibits the production of several cytokines, including IL1, IL6, IL12, tumor necrosis factor-α, and VEGF. There have been reports of activity in iMCD, including a patient with TAFRO syndrome, who had tocilizumab-refractory and prednisone-refractory ascites.[83–86] Other immunomodulatory agents, such as interferon-α and all-trans-retinoic acid, induced complete remissions in incidental cases.[87–90] Although there is rationale for these agents, none has been studied in a systematic fashion and these agents are best reserved for refractory cases or used as adjunctive therapy.

Perhaps more exciting agents are the calcineurin inhibitor cyclosporine and the mammalian target of rapamycin (m-TOR) inhibitor sirolimus. There is emerging evidence that patients with iMCD have activated T-cells and elevated soluble IL2 receptor levels.[91] Cyclosporin binds to cyclophilin and inhibits the phosphatase activity of calcineurin, thereby reducing the release of inflammatory cytokines by T-lymphocytes. Cyclosporin-induced remission in 2 patients with TAFRO syndrome who had failed corticosteroids and tocilizumab and prednisone, respectively.[35,92] Sirolimus inhibits the m-TOR pathway critical to T-cell activation and VEGF secretion. Elevated VEGF levels are common in iMCD and resolve with successful anti-IL6 mAb therapy. Furthermore, high VEGF levels are also frequently seen in POEMS. However, some patients with iMCD fail tocilizumab or siltuximab, and in 1 patient, an extended remission for more than 39 months was maintained with sirolimus and intravenous immunoglobulin after reinduction of combination chemotherapy. Sirolimus is an interesting agent that deserves further investigation in the therapy of iMCD either during remission induction or as maintenance strategy.

Treatment Guidelines and Algorithm

The treatment algorithm depicted in **Fig. 2** outlines a practical approach to the therapy of iMCD. It is critical to select the appropriate therapy for individual patients. More severely ill patients will typically have more marked B-symptoms, thrombocytopenia rather than thrombocytosis, renal dysfunction or other organ dysfunction, and clinical evidence of vascular leak syndrome with ascites and or/pleural effusions. On the other end of the spectrum, some patients have few clinical symptoms and minor findings in terms of abnormal physical examination or laboratory values.

In one study, 60% of patients did not receive siltuximab as front-line therapy and, as previously stated, there may be a bias toward using rituximab.[40] How does one decide to start with rituximab or anti-IL6 mAb (tocilizumab or siltuximab)? In the randomized Phase II siltuximab study, CR and PR were seen in only 34% of patients, although more than 50% remained on study. This study may have enrolled patients who were less sick due to presence of a placebo arm in which patients at best could receive prednisone at a maximum dose of 1 mg/kg. Furthermore, there were stringently defined failure criteria, which may have not allowed some patients time to

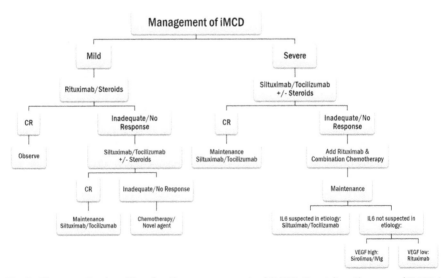

Fig. 2. Therapeutic algorithm for the management of iMCD. Front-line therapy of iMCD is determined by disease severity at presentation. Further modifications to treatment strategy are dependent on response to front-line approach and clinical features.

respond. In contrast, Nishimoto and colleagues[93] reported a continued response rate of 86% to tocilizumab with more than 90% of patients having elevated IL6 levels and all had a clear systemic inflammatory syndrome underscored by abnormal acute phase reactants, anemia, and hypoalbuminemia. A systematic literature review compared baseline of features of patients mostly treated on the siltuximab trials and found less severe clinical and biochemical features in the clinical trial patients.[45] Although numbers were small, the 2-year survival was best in patients treated with anti-IL6 mAbs. Yu and colleagues[40] reported a superior CR rate with siltuximab compared with rituximab-based chemotherapy (43% vs 20%), with a strong trend to superior DFS. The main message from these considerations is that the principal beneficiaries of siltuximab or tocilizumab therapy are patients who are more severely afflicted and have a clear proinflammatory syndrome. It is important to realize that it takes time to respond to anti-IL6 mAb therapy, and induction therapy with siltuximab or tocilizumab is best paired with concomitant steroid therapy, which can later be tapered. Patients who attain a sustained response should be maintained on anti-IL6 mAb therapy and in many, dosing intervals can be expanded.

More severely ill patients who do not respond to IL6 blockade probably comprise 2 patient populations. One group of patients consists of those for whom anti-IL6 agents as sole intervention do not suffice and combination chemotherapy with addition of rituximab may be required to gain control of the disease. There still may be a role for tocilizumab or siltuximab during maintenance. In a second group, IL6 may not be the key driver of the disease and other cytokines and chemokines may play a critical role, which is an active topic of investigation. Preliminary data in 2 patients suggest that the m-TOR pathway is activated in the lymph nodes with TAFRO syndrome and one has used sirolimus to maintain remission (Fajgenbaum personal communication, 2017). Future studies will have to determine whether biomarkers, such as VEGF, can be used to stratify a maintenance approach.

Patients with milder disease are candidates for a more limited treatment approach with 4 to 8 weekly doses of rituximab 375 mg/m^2, which are often combined with steroids. In one study, combination chemotherapy was not superior to rituximab.[40] Rituximab is considerably less toxic and seems therefore a reasonable option for this patient group.[40] Responding patients may not require a maintenance approach. Treatment failures could go on to receive anti-IL6 mAb therapy. Chemotherapy or immunomodulatory agents are best reserved for more refractory patients.

Patients with coexistent POEMS syndrome may require both therapy for POEMS and their iMCD. The progressive sensorimotor polyneuropathy of POEMS does not respond to anti-IL6 mAb therapy. However, anti-IL6 therapy or rituximab may be useful to treat iMCD in patients with both POEMS and iMCD. ASCT is not routinely recommended for iMCD and has been limited to case reports.[94–97] However, patients with coexistent for POEMS syndrome should be considered for ASCT. Some patients with iMCD have features of POEMS (eg, osteosclerotic bone lesions), but do not meet the criteria for the diagnosis of POEMS. Usually these patients do not have a marked proinflammatory syndrome and are preferably managed with rituximab-based therapy as initial intervention.

There are presently no established criteria for measuring response. Ideally, measurement of response should take into account (1) the different manifestations of the disease, which can be broken down into lymphadenopathy/organomegaly, clinical symptomatology, and laboratory parameters; and (2) the kinetics of the response. It is important to recognize that clinical and laboratory parameters often improve more rapidly with anti-IL6 agents, although it takes 6 doses to achieve steady state with siltuximab. In contrast, the involution of lymph nodes with anti-IL6 mAbs occurs at much slower pace than other therapeutic interventions. In this context, it is useful to point out that anti-IL6 mAbs are not lympholytic, but merely neutralize important growth and survival stimuli. These considerations highlight the need for establishing consensus criteria to measure response at well-defined time points, which will facilitate comparisons of future studies.

In clinical practice laboratory markers, such as CRP, erythrocyte sedimentation rate, hemoglobin, and albumin are useful in monitoring response. IL6 levels become uninformative after treatment with tocilizumab and siltuximab due to complexing of IL6 with these drugs leading to falsely elevated IL6 levels. Resolution of lymphadenopathy will be more rapid with chemotherapy and rituximab rather than anti-IL6 mAb therapy. Symptoms and physical findings often also improve rapidly with the exception of symptomatology due to vascular leak syndrome; ascites can be especially persistent, and may take 2 to 3 months to resolve fully.

SUMMARY

Much progress has been made in our understanding of the heterogeneous iMCD disease spectrum, leading to a new classification and diagnostic criteria.[33,98] Anti-IL6 mAbs are an important new tool for the therapy of iMCD and should be considered as front-line therapy for many patients, especially those who are more symptomatic. However, enthusiasm should be tempered by the notion that not all respond and that therapy is not curative. Ultimately, further progress must come from future research elucidating the cause(s) of iMCD, leading to the development of rational and definitive therapies for all patients. Reporting of patients to the CDCN global ACCELERATE registry, which plans to enroll 500 patients over the next 5 years, will permit more comprehensive characterization of the clinical features and natural history of iMCD.[99] A comprehensive real-world analysis of the efficacy of existing therapies will allow for better tailoring of treatments to individual patients in the future.

REFERENCES

1. Castleman B, Towne VW. Case records of the Massachusetts General Hospital; weekly clinicopathological exercises; founded by Richard C. Cabot. N Engl J Med 1954;251(10):396–400.
2. Castleman B, Iverson L, Menendez VP. Localized mediastinal lymph node hyperplasia resembling thymoma. Cancer 1956;9:822–30.
3. Peterson BA, Frizzera G. Multicentric Castleman's disease. Semin Oncol 1993; 20(6):636–47.
4. van Rhee F, Stone K, Szmania S, et al. Castleman disease in the 21st century: an update on diagnosis, assessment, and therapy. Clin Adv Hematol Oncol 2010; 8(7):486–98.
5. Stone K, Woods E, Szmania S, et al. Prevalence of interleukin-6 receptor polymorphism in Castleman disease and association with increased soluble interleukin-6 receptor levels. J Clin Oncol 2011;29 [abstr: 8077].
6. Liu YC, Stone K, van Rhee F. Siltuximab for multicentric Castleman disease. Expert Rev Hematol 2014;7(5):545–57.
7. Hall PA, Donaghy M, Cotter FE, et al. An immunohistological and genotypic study of the plasma cell form of Castleman's disease. Histopathology 1989;14(4): 333–46 [discussion: 429–32].
8. Menke DM, Tiemann M, Camoriano JK, et al. Diagnosis of Castleman's disease by identification of an immunophenotypically aberrant population of mantle

zone B lymphocytes in paraffin-embedded lymph node biopsies. Am J Clin Pathol 1996;105(3):268–76.

9. Sharma S, Nemeth E, Chen YH, et al. Involvement of hepcidin in the anemia of multiple myeloma. Clin Cancer Res 2008;14(11):3262–7.

10. Song SN, Tomosugi N, Kawabata H, et al. Down-regulation of hepcidin resulting from long-term treatment with an anti-IL-6 receptor antibody (tocilizumab) improves anemia of inflammation in multicentric Castleman disease. Blood 2010; 116(18):3627–34.

11. Yoshizaki K, Matsuda T, Nishimoto N, et al. Pathogenic significance of interleukin-6 (IL-6/BSF-2) in Castleman's disease. Blood 1989;74(4):1360–7.

12. Momoi A, Kojima M, Sakai T, et al. IL-6-positive classical Hodgkin's lymphoma co-occurring with plasma cell type of Castleman's disease: report of a case. Int J Hematol 2013;97(2):275–9.

13. Gleason BC, Hornick JL. Inflammatory myofibroblastic tumours: where are we now? J Clin Pathol 2008;61(4):428–37.

14. Brandt SJ, Bodine DM, Dunbar CE, et al. Dysregulated interleukin 6 expression produces a syndrome resembling Castleman's disease in mice. J Clin Invest 1990;86(2):592–9.

15. Brandt SJ, Bodine DM, Dunbar CE, et al. Retroviral-mediated transfer of interleukin-6 into hematopoietic cells of mice results in a syndrome resembling Castleman's disease. Curr Top Microbiol Immunol 1990;166:37–41.

16. Aoki Y, Jaffe ES, Chang Y, et al. Angiogenesis and hematopoiesis induced by Kaposi's sarcoma-associated herpesvirus-encoded interleukin-6. Blood 1999; 93(12):4034–43.

17. Katsume A, Saito H, Yamada Y, et al. Anti-interleukin 6 (IL-6) receptor antibody suppresses Castleman's disease like symptoms emerged in IL-6 transgenic mice. Cytokine 2002;20(6):304–11.

18. Screpanti I, Romani L, Musiani P, et al. Lymphoproliferative disorder and imbalanced T-helper response in C/EBP beta-deficient mice. EMBO J 1995;14(9): 1932–41.

19. Suthaus J, Stuhlmann-Laeisz C, Tompkins VS, et al. HHV-8-encoded viral IL-6 collaborates with mouse IL-6 in the development of multicentric Castleman disease in mice. Blood 2012;119(22):5173–81.

20. van Gameren MM, Willemse PH, Mulder NH, et al. Effects of recombinant human interleukin-6 in cancer patients: a phase I-II study. Blood 1994;84(5):1434–41.

21. Ishiyama T, Nakamura S, Akimoto Y, et al. Immunodeficiency and IL-6 production by peripheral blood monocytes in multicentric Castleman's disease. Br J Haematol 1994;86(3):483–9.

22. Leger-Ravet MB, Peuchmaur M, Devergne O, et al. Interleukin-6 gene expression in Castleman's disease. Blood 1991;78(11):2923–30.

23. Lai YM, Li M, Liu CL, et al. Expression of interleukin-6 and its clinicopathological significance in Castleman's disease. Zhonghua Xue Ye Xue Za Zhi 2013;34(5): 404–8 [in Chinese].

24. Chang KC, Wang YC, Hung LY, et al. Monoclonality and cytogenetic abnormalities in hyaline vascular Castleman disease. Mod Pathol 2014;27(6):823–31.

25. Marcelin AG, Aaron L, Mateus C, et al. Rituximab therapy for HIV-associated Castleman disease. Blood 2003;102(8):2786–8.

26. Hoffmann C, Schmid H, Muller M, et al. Improved outcome with rituximab in patients with HIV-associated multicentric Castleman disease. Blood 2011;118(13): 3499–503.

27. Gerard L, Michot JM, Burcheri S, et al. Rituximab decreases the risk of lymphoma in patients with HIV-associated multicentric Castleman disease. Blood 2012; 119(10):2228–33.
28. Uldrick TS, Polizzotto MN, Aleman K, et al. Rituximab plus liposomal doxorubicin in HIV-infected patients with KSHV-associated multicentric Castleman disease. Blood 2014;124(24):3544–52.
29. Dossier A, Meignin V, Fieschi C, et al. Human herpesvirus 8-related Castleman disease in the absence of HIV infection. Clin Infect Dis 2013;56(6):833–42.
30. Nicoli P, Familiari U, Bosa M, et al. HHV8-positive, HIV-negative multicentric Castleman's disease: early and sustained complete remission with rituximab therapy without reactivation of Kaposi sarcoma. Int J Hematol 2009;90(3):392–6.
31. Marietta M, Pozzi S, Luppi M, et al. Acquired haemophilia in HIV negative, HHV-8 positive multicentric Castleman's disease: a case report. Eur J Haematol 2003; 70(3):181–2.
32. Oksenhendler E, Duarte M, Soulier J, et al. Multicentric Castleman's disease in HIV infection: a clinical and pathological study of 20 patients. AIDS 1996;10(1): 61–7.
33. Fajgenbaum DC, Uldrick TS, Bagg A, et al. International, evidence-based consensus diagnostic criteria for HHV-8-negative/idiopathic multicentric Castleman disease. Blood 2017;129(12):1646–57.
34. Masaki Y, Nakajima A, Iwao H, et al. Japanese variant of multicentric Castleman's disease associated with serositis and thrombocytopenia–a report of two cases: is TAFRO syndrome (Castleman-Kojima disease) a distinct clinicopathological entity? J Clin Exp Hematop 2013;53(1):79–85.
35. Inoue M, Ankou M, Hua J, et al. Complete resolution of TAFRO syndrome (thrombocytopenia, anasarca, fever, reticulin fibrosis and organomegaly) after immunosuppressive therapies using corticosteroids and cyclosporin A: a case report. J Clin Exp Hematop 2013;53(1):95–9.
36. Iwaki N, Sato Y, Takata K, et al. Atypical hyaline vascular-type Castleman's disease with thrombocytopenia, anasarca, fever, and systemic lymphadenopathy. J Clin Exp Hematop 2013;53(1):87–93.
37. Tedesco S, Postacchini L, Manfredi L, et al. Successful treatment of a Caucasian case of multifocal Castleman's disease with TAFRO syndrome with a pathophysiology targeted therapy—a case report. Exp Hematol Oncol 2015;4(1):3.
38. Abdo L, Morin C, Collarino R, et al. First European case of TAFRO syndrome associated with Sjogren disease. Am J Intern Med 2014;2(6):102–5.
39. Iwaki N, Fajgenbaum DC, Nabel CS, et al. Clinicopathologic analysis of TAFRO syndrome demonstrates a distinct subtype of HHV-8-negative multicentric Castleman disease. Am J Hematol 2016;91(2):220–6.
40. Yu L, Tu M, Cortes J, et al. Clinical and pathological characteristics of HIV- and HHV-8-negative Castleman disease. Blood 2017;129(12):1658–68.
41. Dispenzieri A. POEMS syndrome: 2017 update on diagnosis, risk stratification, and management. Am J Hematol 2017;92(8):814–29.
42. van Rhee F, Casper C, Voorhees PM, et al. A phase 2, open-label, multicenter study of the long-term safety of siltuximab (an anti-interleukin-6 monoclonal antibody) in patients with multicentric Castleman disease. Oncotarget 2015;6(30): 30408–19.
43. Dispenzieri A, Armitage JO, Loe MJ, et al. The clinical spectrum of Castleman's disease. Am J Hematol 2012;87(11):997–1002.
44. Talat N, Schulte KM. Castleman's disease: systematic analysis of 416 patients from the literature. Oncologist 2011;16(9):1316–24.

45. Liu AY, Nabel CS, Finkelman BS, et al. Idiopathic multicentric Castleman's disease: a systematic literature review. Lancet Haematol 2016;3(4):e163–75.

46. Talat N, Belgaumkar AP, Schulte KM. Surgery in Castleman's disease: a systematic review of 404 published cases. Ann Surg 2012;255(4):677–84.

47. Herrada J, Cabanillas F, Rice L, et al. The clinical behavior of localized and multicentric Castleman disease. Ann Intern Med 1998;128(8):657–62.

48. Bowne WB, Lewis JJ, Filippa DA, et al. The management of unicentric and multicentric Castleman's disease: a report of 16 cases and a review of the literature. Cancer 1999;85(3):706–17.

49. Lerza R, Castello G, Truini M, et al. Splenectomy induced complete remission in a patient with multicentric Castleman's disease and autoimmune hemolytic anemia. Ann Hematol 1999;78(4):193–6.

50. Chronowski GM, Ha CS, Wilder RB, et al. Treatment of unicentric and multicentric Castleman disease and the role of radiotherapy. Cancer 2001;92(3):670–6.

51. Kessler E. Multicentric giant lymph node hyperplasia. A report of seven cases. Cancer 1985;56(10):2446–51.

52. Weisenburger DD, Nathwani BN, Winberg CD, et al. Multicentric angiofollicular lymph node hyperplasia: a clinicopathologic study of 16 cases. Hum Pathol 1985;16(2):162–72.

53. Frizzera G, Peterson BA, Bayrd ED, et al. A systemic lymphoproliferative disorder with morphologic features of Castleman's disease: clinical findings and clinico-pathologic correlations in 15 patients. J Clin Oncol 1985;3(9):1202–16.

54. Nishimoto N, Kanakura Y, Aozasa K, et al. Humanized anti-interleukin-6 receptor antibody treatment of multicentric Castleman disease. Blood 2005;106(8):2627–32.

55. van Rhee F, Wong RS, Munshi N, et al. Siltuximab for multicentric Castleman's disease: a randomised, double-blind, placebo-controlled trial. Lancet Oncol 2014;15(9):966–74.

56. van Rhee F, Szymonifka J, Anaissie E, et al. Total therapy 3 for multiple myeloma: prognostic implications of cumulative dosing and premature discontinuation of VTD maintenance components, bortezomib, thalidomide, and dexamethasone, relevant to all phases of therapy. Blood 2010;116(8):1220–7.

57. Zhu SH, Yu YH, Zhang Y, et al. Clinical features and outcome of patients with HIV-negative multicentric Castleman's disease treated with combination chemotherapy: a report on 10 patients. Med Oncol 2013;30(1):492.

58. Bower M, Powles T, Williams S, et al. Brief communication: rituximab in HIV-associated multicentric Castleman disease. Ann Intern Med 2007;147(12):836–9.

59. Gerard L, Berezne A, Galicier L, et al. Prospective study of rituximab in chemotherapy-dependent human immunodeficiency virus associated multicentric Castleman's disease: ANRS 117 CastlemaB trial. J Clin Oncol 2007;25(22):3350–6.

60. Bower M, Newsom-Davis T, Naresh K, et al. Clinical features and outcome in HIV-associated multicentric Castleman's disease. J Clin Oncol 2011;29(18):2481–6.

61. Ocio EM, Sanchez-Guijo FM, Diez-Campelo M, et al. Efficacy of rituximab in an aggressive form of multicentric Castleman disease associated with immune phenomena. Am J Hematol 2005;78(4):302–5.

62. Ide M, Ogawa E, Kasagi K, et al. Successful treatment of multicentric Castleman's disease with bilateral orbital tumour using rituximab. Br J Haematol 2003;121(5):818–9.

63. Gholam D, Vantelon JM, Al-Jijakli A, et al. A case of multicentric Castleman's disease associated with advanced systemic amyloidosis treated with chemotherapy and anti-CD20 monoclonal antibody. Ann Hematol 2003;82(12):766–8.
64. Beck JT, Hsu SM, Wijdenes J, et al. Brief report: alleviation of systemic manifestations of Castleman's disease by monoclonal anti-interleukin-6 antibody. N Engl J Med 1994;330(9):602–5.
65. Sato K, Tsuchiya M, Saldanha J, et al. Reshaping a human antibody to inhibit the interleukin 6-dependent tumor cell growth. Cancer Res 1993;53(4):851–6.
66. Nishimoto N, Sasai M, Shima Y, et al. Improvement in Castleman's disease by humanized anti-interleukin-6 receptor antibody therapy. Blood 2000;95(1):56–61.
67. Nishimoto N, Honda O, Sumikawa H, et al. A long-term (5-year) sustained efficacy of Tocilizuman for multicentric Castleman's disease and the effect on pulmonary complications. Blood 2007;110.
68. Kawabata H, Kadowaki N, Nishikori M, et al. Clinical features and treatment of multicentric Castleman's disease : a retrospective study of 21 Japanese patients at a single institute. J Clin Exp Hematop 2013;53(1):69–77.
69. Matsuyama M, Suzuki T, Tsuboi H, et al. Anti-interleukin-6 receptor antibody (tocilizumab) treatment of multicentric Castleman's disease. Intern Med 2007; 46(11):771–4.
70. Nagao A, Nakazawa S, Hanabusa H. Short-term efficacy of the IL6 receptor antibody tocilizumab in patients with HIV-associated multicentric Castleman disease: report of two cases. J Hematol Oncol 2014;7:10.
71. Galeotti C, Boucheron A, Guillaume S, et al. Sustained remission of multicentric Castleman disease in children treated with tocilizumab, an anti-interleukin-6 receptor antibody. Mol Cancer Ther 2012;11(8):1623–6.
72. Ding C, Jones G. Anti-interleukin-6 receptor antibody treatment in inflammatory autoimmune diseases. Rev Recent Clin Trials 2006;1(3):193–200.
73. van Rhee F, Fayad L, Voorhees P, et al. Siltuximab, a novel anti-interleukin-6 monoclonal antibody, for Castleman's disease. J Clin Oncol 2010;28(23):3701–8.
74. Kurzrock R, Voorhees PM, Casper C, et al. A phase I, open-label study of siltuximab, an anti-IL-6 monoclonal antibody, in patients with B-cell non-Hodgkin lymphoma, multiple myeloma, or Castleman disease. Clin Cancer Res 2013;19(13):3659–70.
75. Casper C, Chaturvedi S, Munshi N, et al. Analysis of inflammatory and anemia-related biomarkers in a randomized, double-blind, placebo-controlled study of Siltuximab (anti-IL6 monoclonal antibody) in patients with multicentric Castleman disease. Clin Cancer Res 2015;21(19):4294–304.
76. van Rhee F, Rothman M, Ho KF, et al. Patient-reported outcomes for multicentric Castleman's disease in a randomized, placebo-controlled study of siltuximab. Patient 2015;8(2):207–16.
77. Kirk M, Kurzrock R, van Rhee F, et al. Siltuximab reverses muscle wasting in patients with multicentric Castleman's disease. Blood 2013;122(21).
78. Galeotti C, Tran TA, Franchi-Abella S, et al. IL-1RA agonist (anakinra) in the treatment of multifocal Castleman disease: case report. J Pediatr Hematol Oncol 2008;30(12):920–4.
79. El-Osta H, Janku F, Kurzrock R. Successful treatment of Castleman's disease with interleukin-1 receptor antagonist (Anakinra). Mol Cancer Ther 2010;9(6):1485–8.
80. Lin Q, Fang B, Huang H, et al. Efficacy of bortezomib and thalidomide in the recrudescent form of multicentric mixed-type Castleman's disease. Blood Cancer J 2015;5:e298.

81. Hess G, Wagner V, Kreft A, et al. Effects of bortezomib on pro-inflammatory cytokine levels and transfusion dependency in a patient with multicentric Castleman disease. Br J Haematol 2006;134(5):544–5.
82. Yuan ZG, Dun XY, Li YH, et al. Treatment of multicentric Castleman's disease accompanying multiple myeloma with bortezomib: a case report. J Hematol Oncol 2009;2:19.
83. Starkey CR, Joste NE, Lee FC. Near-total resolution of multicentric Castleman disease by prolonged treatment with thalidomide. Am J Hematol 2006;81(4):303–4.
84. Lee FC, Merchant SH. Alleviation of systemic manifestations of multicentric Castleman's disease by thalidomide. Am J Hematol 2003;73(1):48–53.
85. Tatekawa S, Umemura K, Fukuyama R, et al. Thalidomide for tocilizumab-resistant ascites with TAFRO syndrome. Clin Case Rep 2015;3(6):472–8.
86. Ramasamy K, Gandhi S, Tenant-Flowers M, et al. Rituximab and thalidomide combination therapy for Castleman disease. Br J Haematol 2012;158(3):421–3.
87. Tamayo M, Gonzalez C, Majado MJ, et al. Long-term complete remission after interferon treatment in a case of multicentric Castelman's disease. Am J Hematol 1995;49(4):359–60.
88. Simko R, Nagy K, Lombay B, et al. Multicentric Castleman disease and systemic lupus erythematosus phenotype in a boy with Klinefelter syndrome: long-term disease stabilization with interferon therapy. J Pediatr Hematol Oncol 2000; 22(2):180–3.
89. Andres E, Maloisel F. Interferon-alpha as first-line therapy for treatment of multicentric Castleman's disease. Ann Oncol 2000;11(12):1613–4.
90. Rieu P, Droz D, Gessain A, et al. Retinoic acid for treatment of multicentric Castleman's disease. Lancet 1999;354(9186):1262–3.
91. Kawabata H, Takai K, Kojima M, et al. Castleman-Kojima disease (TAFRO syndrome): a novel systemic inflammatory disease characterized by a constellation of symptoms, namely, thrombocytopenia, ascites (anasarca), microcytic anemia, myelofibrosis, renal dysfunction, and organomegaly : a status report and summary of Fukushima (6 June, 2012) and Nagoya meetings (22 September, 2012). J Clin Exp Hematop 2013;53(1):57–61.
92. Yamaga Y, Tokuyama K, Kato T, et al. Successful treatment with cyclosporin A in tocilizumab-resistant TAFRO syndrome. Intern Med 2016;55(2):185–90.
93. Nishimoto N, Honda O, Sumikawa H, et al. A long-term (5 year) sustained efficacy of tocilizumab for multicentric Castleman's disease and the effect on pulmonary complications. ASH Annual Meeting Abstracts. Atlanta (GA), December 8–11, 2007.
94. Tal Y, Haber G, Cohen MJ, et al. Autologous stem cell transplantation in a rare multicentric Castleman disease of the plasma cell variant. Int J Hematol 2011; 93(5):677–80.
95. Repetto L, Jaiprakash MP, Selby PJ, et al. Aggressive angiofollicular lymph node hyperplasia (Castleman's disease) treated with high dose melphalan and autologous bone marrow transplantation. Hematol Oncol 1986;4(3):213–7.
96. Ogita M, Hoshino J, Sogawa Y, et al. Multicentric Castleman disease with secondary AA renal amyloidosis, nephrotic syndrome and chronic renal failure, remission after high-dose melphalan and autologous stem cell transplantation. Clin Nephrol 2007;68(3):171–6.
97. Advani R, Warnke R, Rosenberg S. Treatment of multicentric Castleman's disease complicated by the development of non-Hodgkin's lymphoma with high-dose chemotherapy and autologous peripheral stem-cell support. Ann Oncol 1999; 10(10):1207–9.

98. Fajgenbaum DC, van Rhee F, Nabel CS. HHV-8-negative, idiopathic multicentric Castleman disease: novel insights into biology, pathogenesis, and therapy. Blood 2014;123(19):2924–33.

99. Fajgenbaum DC, Ruth JR, Kelleher D, et al. The collaborative network approach: a new framework to accelerate Castleman's disease and other rare disease research. Lancet Haematol 2016;3(4):e150–2.

TAFRO Syndrome

Takuro Igawa, MD[a], Yasuharu Sato, MD[a,b],*

KEYWORDS

- TAFRO syndrome • Castleman disease • Clinical features • Pathogenesis

KEY POINTS

- TAFRO syndrome is a newly recognized variant of idiopathic multicentric Castleman disease (iMCD) that involves a constellation of syndromes: thrombocytopenia (T), anasarca (A), fever (F), reticulin fibrosis (R), and organomegaly (O).
- Thrombocytopenia and severe anasarca accompanied by relatively low serum immunoglobulin levels are characteristic clinical findings of TAFRO syndrome that are not present in iMCD–not otherwise specified (iMCD-NOS).
- Lymph node biopsy is recommended to exclude other diseases and to diagnose TAFRO syndrome, which reveals characteristic histopathological findings similar to hyaline vascular-type Castleman disease.
- TAFRO syndrome takes a more aggressive course than iMCD-NOS.
- The main therapeutic options include corticosteroids, immunosuppressive therapy (eg, cyclosporin A), rituximab or rituximab-based therapy, and anti-interleukin-6 therapies (eg, tocilizumab and siltuximab).

INTRODUCTION

TAFRO syndrome is a recently recognized systemic disease that was initially identified by Takai and colleagues in 2010.[1] The investigators reported 3 cases that shared characteristic clinical symptoms, which included thrombocytopenia (T), anasarca (A), fever (F), reticulin fibrosis (R), and organomegaly (O).[1] Only 1 of the 3 patients underwent lymph node biopsy, and the specimen exhibited histologic features similar to those of Castleman disease (CD). Thus, Takai and colleagues suggested that TAFRO syndrome might be a unique variant of CD.

Disclosure: The authors have no conflict of interest to disclosure.
This work was partially supported by a Grant-in-Aid for Scientific Research (C) (JSPS KAKENHI Grant Number JP16K08666) from the Japan Society for the Promotion of Science.
[a] Department of Pathology, Okayama University Graduate School of Medicine, Dentistry and Pharmaceutical Sciences, 2-5-1 Shikata-cho, Kita-ku, Okayama 700-8558, Japan; [b] Division of Pathophysiology, Okayama University Graduate School of Health Sciences, 2-5-1 Shikata-cho, Kita-ku, Okayama 700-8558, Japan
* Corresponding author. Division of Pathophysiology, Okayama University Graduate School of Health Sciences, 2-5-1 Shikata-cho, Kita-ku, Okayama 700-8558, Japan.
E-mail address: satou-y@okayama-u.ac.jp

Hematol Oncol Clin N Am 32 (2018) 107–118
https://doi.org/10.1016/j.hoc.2017.09.009
0889-8588/18/© 2017 Elsevier Inc. All rights reserved.

CD is a rare and poorly understood lymphoproliferative disorder that was originally described by Castleman and colleagues in 1956.[2] This disorder consists of heterogeneous diseases that share several histopathological findings, and can be histologically divided into hyaline vascular (HV)-type or plasma cell (PC)-type CD.[3] Cases of HV-type CD exhibit interfollicular vascular proliferation that often penetrates the atrophic germinal centers, whereas PC-type CD generally exhibits expanded intrafollicular areas with sheets of mature plasma cells.[4,5] The germinal centers of PC-type CD can be hyperplastic or atrophic, and the hyalinized vessels and follicular dendritic cell dysplasia that are seen in HV-type CD are not observed in PC-type CD.[4,6] However, HV-type CD also exhibits findings that are characteristic of PC-type CD and vice versa.[4,7] The overlapping features of CD sometimes make it difficult to differentiate between the 2 histologic types, and these cases are referred to as mixed-type CD.[4,7]

CD cases that involve solitary or multiple lymph node regions are classified as unicentric CD (UCD) and multicentric CD (MCD), respectively.[4,8] Patients with UCD typically have a single asymptomatic enlarged lymph node with histologic features of HV-type CD, whereas patients with MCD present with multifocal lymph node swelling and histologic features of PC-type CD.[5,7,9] HV-type CD features are also observed in cases of MCD.[7,9] Patients with MCD experience a more progressive course, compared with patients with UCD, and MCD cases are accompanied by systemic manifestations, such as fever with abnormal laboratory findings (eg, anemia, thrombocytosis, polyclonal hypergammaglobulinemia, and elevated acute phase protein levels).[7,9]

As CD is defined according to common histopathological findings, it includes heterogeneous disorders with overlapping clinicopathological manifestations. It is now understood that MCD encompasses a heterogeneous group of systemic inflammatory disorders caused by hypercytokinemia (ie, involving interleukin [IL]-6).[4,9] Human herpes virus (HHV)-8 is a known etiologic agent that causes MCD by producing a viral homolog of IL-6, especially in immunocompromised cases (eg, patients who are infected with the human immunodeficiency virus).[10,11] To date, the etiology of non–HHV-8 MCD has remained unknown, with these cases collectively referred to as idiopathic MCD (iMCD) **(Fig. 1)**.[12] MCD in Western countries was often thought to be caused

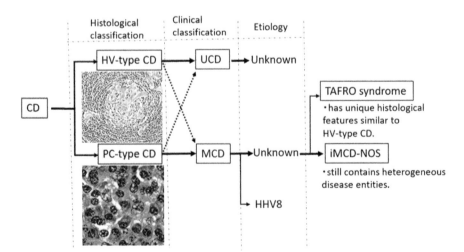

Fig. 1. Relationship between CD and TAFRO syndrome.

by HHV-8,[5] until Fajgenbaum and colleagues[12] demonstrated in 2014 that iMCD is also prevalent and accounts for more than 50% of all American MCD cases. In contrast, almost all Japanese MCD cases are negative for HHV-8.[13] Thus, iMCD is expected to represent a distinct condition with dysregulated cytokine activity and a different pathogenesis.

In this context, Takai and colleagues[1] suggested in 2010 that TAFRO syndrome was a variant of iMCD. In our previous study in 2016, we reported that TAFRO syndrome may represent a distinct subtype of iMCD that shares some clinical and histologic characteristics based on the findings of 25 TAFRO syndrome cases (including 2 Westerners) and 19 non-TAFRO iMCD cases (iMCD–not otherwise specified [iMCD-NOS]).[14] Many reports have described TAFRO syndrome in Japan and other countries, and this disease entity is becoming broadly appreciated.[15–22] The subclassification of iMCD may provide beneficial information regarding prognosis, treatments, and novel therapeutic targets.

Patients with unidentified TAFRO syndrome may have been reported in the literature. For example, before TAFRO syndrome was identified in 2010, Kojima and colleagues[23] had classified Japanese MCD cases into 2 types: an idiopathic plasmacytic lymphadenopathy with polyclonal hyperimmunoglobulinemia (IPL)-type and a non-IPL type. A retrospective analysis of their findings suggests that the non-IPL type MCD shares clinicopathological characteristics in common with TAFRO syndrome. Hence, some reports have described TAFRO syndrome as Castleman-Kojima disease.[24–26]

This review aimed to describe this newly recognized disease entity, including its clinicopathological characteristics, diagnostic challenges, and treatment options.

CLINICAL CHARACTERISTICS
Age at Onset

The median age of patients with TAFRO syndrome is reportedly 50 to 59 years old, and there is no difference between male and female patients.[14,21] A few young patients (14–22 years old) have been reported.[25,27,28]

Symptoms

TAFRO syndrome follows an acute or subacute clinical course.[14,21] The median time from its onset to lymph node biopsy is 6 weeks, which is shorter than the interval for iMCD-NOS.[14] Patients with TAFRO syndrome have a poor general condition at their diagnosis, with a typical Eastern Cooperative Oncology Group performance status of $\geq$2.[14] In addition, patients with TAFRO syndrome exhibit fever without obvious infection (61.1%–84.0%) and severe anasarca (96%–100%).[14,21] Massive pleural effusion and/or ascites are frequently observed, and many patients have organomegaly (88.9%–100%), which typically includes mild lymph node swelling, hepatomegaly, or splenomegaly.[14,21] Some patients have painful lymph node swelling.[14] Uptake of ^{18}F-fluorodeoxyglucose in the swollen organs is only slightly elevated during positron emission tomography.[22] Some patients with TAFRO syndrome have abdominal pain at disease onset (32%),[14] and TAFRO syndrome can involve progressive acute kidney failure that requires transient hemodialysis.[14,21]

Laboratory Findings

Thrombocytopenia and relatively low serum gamma globulin levels are characteristic laboratory findings that can be used to distinguish between TAFRO syndrome and iMCD-NOS.[14,21] In cases of TAFRO syndrome, the median platelet count is 43,000/μL and the median serum immunoglobulin (Ig)G level is 1476 mg/dL.[14] One series of 18 Japanese patients with TAFRO syndrome revealed that all patients had thrombocytopenia (<100,000/μL).[21] Serum alkaline phosphatase (ALP) levels are elevated in 64.3% to 79.2% of patients with TAFRO syndrome, although there are no corresponding elevations in transaminase levels.[14,21] Other laboratory findings from patients with TAFRO syndrome include anemia, hypoalbuminemia, and elevated levels of serum C-reactive protein and soluble IL-2 receptor.[14,21] Serum creatinine levels in TAFRO syndrome cases range from 0.52 mg/dL to 6.08 mg/dL (median, 0.96 mg/dL).[14] Serum lactate dehydrogenase levels are not elevated in TAFRO syndrome.[14] Serum IL-6 levels at the diagnosis of TAFRO syndrome exhibit a milder elevation, compared with iMCD-NOS, although there appears to be no statistically significant difference.[14,21] Serum levels of vascular endothelial growth factor are elevated in TAFRO syndrome.[14,21]

HISTOPATHOLOGICAL CHARACTERISTICS
Lymph Nodes

Patients with TAFRO syndrome have slightly enlarged lymph nodes, with a greatest diameter that ranges from 6 mm to 14 mm (median, 9 mm).[14] Some histologic findings of TAFRO syndrome are unique, compared with iMCD-NOS, although both disorders also share some histologic features.[14] Lymph node specimens from patients with TAFRO syndrome exhibit atrophic germinal centers with expanded interfollicular areas (**Fig. 2**). Marked proliferation of high endothelial venules with relatively small numbers of mature plasma cells is observed in the interfollicular areas. Immunostaining for CD21 can reveal expanded or disrupted follicular dendritic cell networks. Blood vessels that penetrate the follicles are present, but inconspicuous. These findings are features of HV-type CD, although lymph node specimens from patients with TAFRO syndrome do not have other features of HV-type CD (eg, hyalinized blood vessels). The endothelial cells in the germinal centers and interfollicular areas have conspicuously enlarged nuclei, a finding that differs from HV-type CD. Light chain restrictions are not observed using in situ hybridization, and HHV-8 infection is not detected using immunostaining for latency-associated nuclear antigen-1.

Bone Marrow

Bone marrow specimens from patients with TAFRO syndrome tend to exhibit hypercellular marrow with megakaryocytic hyperplasia (**Fig. 3**),[14] although approximately 10% of cases exhibit hypocellular marrow.[14] Specimens also exhibit megakaryocytes with slight atypia, such as multiple and widely separated nuclei, and plasma cell infiltration is not prominent. Silver staining reveals reticulin fibrosis in 75.0% to 81.3% of TAFRO syndrome cases (see **Fig. 3**), with a very loose network of reticulin fibers. In some instances, bone marrow cannot be obtained through aspiration (the "dry tap").

DIAGNOSIS
The Need for Differential Diagnosis

Although TAFRO syndrome and iMCD-NOS share some clinical and pathologic features, several distinct clinicopathological findings can be used to differentiate between the 2 conditions (**Fig. 4**). HHV-8–positive MCD can be easily diagnosed by detecting latency-associated nuclear antigen-1–positive cells in lymph node biopsy specimens.[10,29]

As there are no known specific markers for diagnosing TAFRO syndrome, the diagnosis must exclude other diseases that mimic TAFRO syndrome, such as infectious diseases, autoimmune diseases, and malignancy. For example, angioimmunoblastic T-cell lymphoma may present with severe anasarca, and the diagnosis must exclude

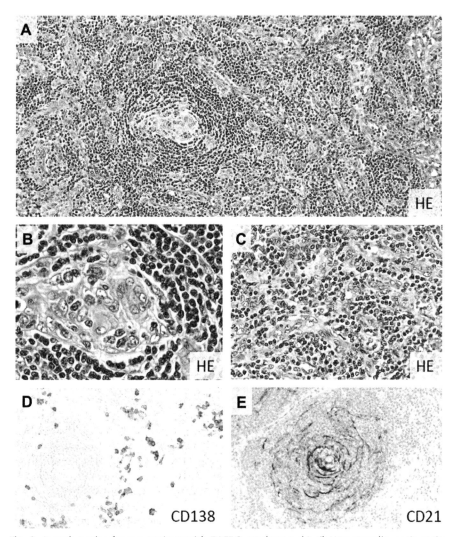

Fig. 2. Lymph nodes from a patient with TAFRO syndrome. (*A–C*) Hematoxylin-eosin stain-ing; (*D*) CD138 immunostaining; (*E*) CD21 immunostaining. (*A*) A mildly enlarged lymph node exhibits atrophic germinal centers and marked proliferation of high endothelial venules in the germinal centers and expanded interfollicular areas. (*B*) The germinal centers do not contain hyalinized penetrating blood vessels, and the nuclei of the proliferating endothelial cells are prominently enlarged. (*C, D*) Unlike plasma cell-type Castleman disease, the plasma cell infiltration in the interfollicular area is not conspicuous. (*E*) CD21 immuno-staining highlights the expanded follicular dendritic cell networks.

this condition in the absence of accompanying hypergammaglobulinemia.[30,31] A similar exclusion process is needed for iMCD-NOS.[4]

Proposed Diagnostic Criteria

After ruling out diseases that mimic TAFRO syndrome, the diagnosis of TAFRO syn-drome should be established based on a combination of the clinical and histopatho-logical findings. We have previously proposed diagnostic criteria for TAFRO syndrome

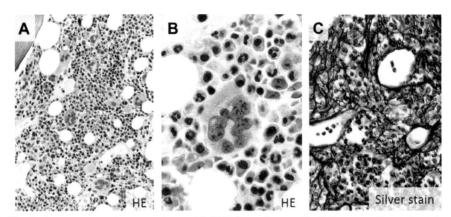

Fig. 3. Bone marrow from a patient with TAFRO syndrome. (*A, B*) Hematoxylin-eosin staining; (*C*) Silver staining. (*A*) Hypercellular marrow is observed with hyperplastic megakaryocytes. (*B*) The megakaryocytes have slight atypia with widely separated nuclei. (*C*) Silver staining reveals a very loose network of reticulin fibers.

(**Box 1**).[14] These criteria require histologic findings from a lymph node biopsy specimen that are compatible with TAFRO syndrome, as well as 3 to 5 TAFRO syndromes being present (thrombocytopenia, anasarca, fever, reticulin fibrosis, and organomegaly), the absence of hypergammaglobulinemia, and small-volume lymphadenopathy. In addition, patients should fulfill at least 1 of the minor criteria: hyperplasia/

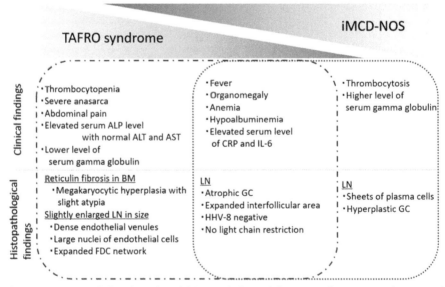

Fig. 4. Summary of the clinical and histopathological features of TAFRO syndrome and iMCD-NOS. Although TAFRO syndrome and iMCD-NOS have clinicopathological features in common, TAFRO syndrome has unique characteristics that can distinguish it from iMCD-NOS. ALT, alanine transaminase; AST, aspartate transaminase; BM, bone marrow; CRP, C-reactive protein; FDC, follicular dendritic cell; GC, germinal center; LN, lymph node; NOS, not otherwise specified.

Box 1
Proposed diagnostic criteria for TAFRO syndrome

Differential diagnosis is essential from other disorders
- Autoimmune/autoinflammatory diseases; SLE, RA, Still disease
- Infectious diseases; eg, EBV infection, HIV infection
- Neoplastic diseases; eg, AITL, POEMS syndrome

1. Histopathological criteria (need both)
   - Compatible with histopathological findings of lymph nodes as TAFRO syndrome
   - Negative LANA-1 for HHV-8

2. Major criteria (need all)
   - Presents at least 3 of 5 TAFRO symptoms
     i. Thrombocytopenia
     ii. Anasarca
     iii. Fever
     iv. Reticulin fibrosis
     v. Organomegaly
   - Absence of hypergammaglobulinemia
   - Small-volume lymphadenopathy

3. Minor criteria (need 1 or more)
   - Hyper/normoplasia of megakaryocytes in bone marrow
   - High levels of serum ALP without markedly elevated serum transaminase

Abbreviations: AITL, angioimmunoblastic T-cell lymphoma; ALP, alkaline phosphatase; EBV, Epstein-Barr virus; HHV-8, human herpesvirus 8; HIV, human immunodeficiency virus; LANA, latency-associated nuclear antigen; POEMS, polyneuropathy, organomegaly, endocrinopathy, monoclonal gammopathy, and skin changes; RA, rheumatoid arthritis; SLE, systemic lupus erythematosus; TAFRO, thrombocytopenia (T); anasarca (A), fever (F), reticulin fibrosis (R), and organomegaly (O).
   Adapted from Iwaki N, Fajgenbaum DC, Nabel CS, et al. Clinicopathologic analysis of TAFRO syndrome demonstrates a distinct subtype of HHV-8-negative multicentric Castleman disease. Am J Hematol 2016;91(2):225; with permission.

---

normoplasia of megakaryocytes in the bone marrow and high serum ALP levels without elevated serum transaminase levels. For these criteria, thrombocytopenia is defined as a platelet count of less than 100,000/μL, fever is defined as a temperature of greater than 38.0°C (>100.4°F), anasarca is defined as the presence of pleural fluids and ascites during computed tomography, and organomegaly is defined as the presence of lymphadenopathy, hepatomegaly, or splenomegaly.

Importance of Lymph Node Biopsy

Masaki and colleagues[21] have published diagnostic criteria for TAFRO syndrome that do not essentially require lymph node biopsy. These criteria require the presence of anasarca, thrombocytopenia, and systemic inflammation, as well as the fulfillment of at least 2 of the 4 minor criteria: CD-like findings from lymph node biopsy, reticulin myelofibrosis, and/or an increased number of megakaryocytes in the bone marrow, mild organomegaly, and progressive renal insufficiency. However, relying exclusively on clinical symptoms can lead to the misdiagnosis of TAFRO syndrome, and it remains important to exclude autoimmune disease, infectious disease, and malignancy using histologic specimens.

PROGNOSIS AND CLASSIFICATION OF SEVERITY

A recent retrospective cohort study revealed that TAFRO syndrome is associated with inferior survival, compared with iMCD-NOS.[9] The disease activity of cases with

TAFRO syndrome tends to be high during the initial clinical phase, which can lead to mortality caused by disease progression and/or infection in 11.1% to 12.0% of cases.[14,21] No cases of malignancy secondary to TAFRO syndrome have been reported.[14]

Masaki and colleagues[21] proposed a system for grading the severity of TAFRO syndrome, with maximum scores of 3 points calculated for anasarca, platelet depletion, fever and/or inflammation, and renal dysfunction. These subscores are added and the total score is used to classify disease severity as ranging from Grade 1 (3–4 points) to Grade 5 (11–12 points). That study evaluated 18 patients with TAFRO syndrome who were classified as having Grade 1 (5.5%), Grade 2 (61.1%), Grade 3 (22.2%), Grade 4 (11.1%), and Grade 5 (0%) disease.

DISEASE MECHANISMS
The Role of Interleukin-6

Although little is known regarding the etiology and pathophysiology of TAFRO syndrome, the involved syndromes must be related to hypercytokinemia. IL-6 is a multifunctional cytokine that elicits a broad range of cellular and physiologic responses that can lead to varied symptoms, including fever, anemia, and increased immunoglobulin and platelet production.[12] Although IL-6 is considered a major proinflammatory cytokine in the pathophysiology of iMCD-NOS, IL-6 does not appear to be a major pathogenic cytokine in TAFRO syndrome, because the clinical features of TAFRO syndrome lack some symptoms that are associated with IL-6 (eg, thrombocytosis and polyclonal hypergammaglobulinemia). Cytokines other than IL-6 may play an important role in the pathophysiology of TAFRO syndrome, although it is associated with mildly elevated serum IL-6 levels. Severe anasarca may be caused by its unique cytokine profile.

Platelet Count Depletion

Thrombocytopenia and hypercellular bone marrow with megakaryocytic hyperplasia are characteristic manifestations of TAFRO syndrome.[14] The bone marrow findings suggest that platelets undergo extramedullary consumption or destruction. Immune-mediated accelerated platelet destruction, the characteristic pathogenic hallmark of immune thrombocytopenia, may be involved in the thrombocytopenia associated with TAFRO syndrome. In fact, in the report by Takai and colleagues in 2010,[1] platelet-associated IgG levels were elevated in patients with TAFRO syndrome, including 1 patient who was positive for anti-GPIIb/IIIa antibodies. Splenomegaly in TAFRO syndrome may arise from platelet destruction in the spleen. The significance of reticulin fibrosis in TAFRO syndrome is largely unknown.

Is Bacterial Infection a Cause of TAFRO Syndrome?

Recent research has analyzed the cytokine profiles of patients with TAFRO syndrome, and revealed that they had elevated serum levels of interferon-γ induced protein-10 (IP-10), compared with patients with iMCD-NOS and healthy controls.[32] Elevated levels of IP-10 are associated with autoinflammatory mechanisms as well as viral and bacterial infections.[33,34] Serum procalcitonin levels have also been reported to be elevated in patients with TAFRO syndrome,[32,35] which are closely associated with bacterial infections.[36] Therefore, bacterial infections may be involved in the pathogenesis of TAFRO syndrome. Because increased serum IP-10 and procalcitonin levels are not accompanied by elevated levels of interferon-gamma,[32] it seems unlikely that a virus is involved in the pathogenesis of TAFRO syndrome, although a non–HHV-8 virus is considered a possible cause of iMCD-NOS.[12] Interestingly, some patients with TAFRO syndrome experience abdominal pain that coincides with elevations in serum ALP levels, which is not accompanied by corresponding elevations in transaminase levels.[14] These unique findings suggest that TAFRO syndrome might be triggered by bile duct infection, resulting in systemic immunologic abnormalities. A report of a Japanese patient with TAFRO syndrome described neutrophil infiltration in the portal area of the liver.[37] This should have been considered as nonspecific inflammation in the previous reports of TAFRO syndrome that included findings from liver biopsy.[25,27,38] Further studies are needed to better understand the etiology and pathophysiology of TAFRO syndrome.

CLINICAL MANAGEMENT

No standard treatment is available for TAFRO syndrome. The main therapeutic options include corticosteroids, immunosuppressive therapy (eg, cyclosporin A), rituximab or rituximab-based therapy, and anti-IL-6 therapies (eg, tocilizumab and siltuximab).[9,21] In 2 Japanese series of TAFRO syndrome cases, almost all patients initially received corticosteroids (eg, prednisolone, methylprednisolone, and dexamethasone).[14,21] In 1 series of 25 Japanese patients with TAFRO syndrome, 47.8% of patients responded well to corticosteroid therapy, although some refractory cases required additional therapeutic interventions (eg, cyclosporin A, tocilizumab, or rituximab) and 3 patients died (2 of disease progression and 1 of sepsis).[14] Some patients with severe renal dysfunction require temporary dialysis during flare-ups, and plasma exchange is also needed in severe cases. Masaki and colleagues[21] have proposed a treatment strategy for TAFRO syndrome that involves initial treatment using high-dose prednisolone (1 mg/kg per day for 2 weeks) with tapering or methyl-prednisolone pulse therapy (500–1000 mg/d for 3 days) in emergent cases. Nevertheless, this approach requires prospective investigation, as it was based on experience with a relatively small number of cases.

   In contrast to Japan, siltuximab has been approved for use in North America, Europe, and Brazil.[39] Siltuximab effectively blocks the IL-6 signaling pathway and controls various clinical symptoms and laboratory findings in patients with iMCD.[40,41] A recent report described 43 patients with iMCD, including 9 patients with TAFRO variants, and revealed that siltuximab could provide a better complete response rate for the TAFRO variants compared with chemotherapy or corticosteroids.[9] The investigators recommended using siltuximab as the first-line treatment for iMCD and TAFRO syndrome, with the addition of corticosteroids to relieve any acute symptoms.[9] However, as IL-6 does not appear to be a major pathogenic driver of TAFRO syndrome, more specific treatments may be required, especially because anti-IL-6 therapies can lead to relapse if the therapy is terminated.[9,42]

SUMMARY

TAFRO syndrome is a newly recognized variant of iMCD that involves a constellation of symptoms: thrombocytopenia (T), anasarca (A), fever (F), reticulin fibrosis (R), and organomegaly (O). Thrombocytopenia and severe anasarca in the absence of polyclonal hypergammaglobulinemia are distinct clinical features of TAFRO syndrome, which distinguish it from iMCD-NOS. TAFRO syndrome also exhibits characteristic histopathological findings that resemble HV-type CD. Although TAFRO syndrome is now understood to be a variant of iMCD, further studies are needed to elucidate the etiology of TAFRO syndrome and to better differentiate it from iMCD.

REFERENCES

1. Takai K, Nikkuni K, Shibuya H, et al. Thrombocytopenia with mild bone marrow fibrosis accompanied by fever, pleural effusion, ascites and hepatosplenomegaly. Rinsho ketsueki 2010;51(5):320–5.
2. Castleman B, Iverson L, Menendez VP. Localized mediastinal lymph node hyperplasia resembling thymoma. Cancer 1956;9(4):822–30.
3. Keller AR, Hochholzer L, Castleman B. Hyaline-vascular and plasma-cell types of giant lymph node hyperplasia of the mediastinum and other locations. Cancer 1972;29(3):670–83.
4. Fajgenbaum DC, Uldrick TS, Bagg A, et al. International, evidence-based consensus diagnostic criteria for HHV-8-negative/idiopathic multicentric Castleman disease. Blood 2017;129(12):1646–57.
5. Waterston A, Bower M. Fifty years of multicentric Castleman's disease. Acta Oncol 2004;43(8):698–704.
6. Sato Y, Kojima M, Takata K, et al. Multicentric Castleman's disease with abundant IgG4-positive cells: a clinical and pathological analysis of six cases. J Clin Pathol 2010;63(12):1084–9.
7. Dispenzieri A, Armitage JO, Loe MJ, et al. The clinical spectrum of Castleman's disease. Am J Hematol 2012;87(11):997–1002.
8. Frizzera G, Peterson BA, Bayrd ED, et al. A systemic lymphoproliferative disorder with morphologic features of Castleman's disease: clinical findings and clinicopathologic correlations in 15 patients. J Clin Oncol 1985;3(9):1202–16.
9. Yu L, Tu M, Cortes J, et al. Clinical and pathological characteristics of HIV- and HHV-8-negative Castleman disease. Blood 2017;129(12):1658–68.
10. Dupin N, Diss TL, Kellam P, et al. HHV-8 is associated with a plasmablastic variant of Castleman disease that is linked to HHV-8-positive plasmablastic lymphoma. Blood 2000;95(4):1406–12.
11. Aoki Y, Jaffe ES, Chang Y, et al. Angiogenesis and hematopoiesis induced by Kaposi's sarcoma-associated herpesvirus-encoded interleukin-6. Blood 1999;93(12):4034–43.
12. Fajgenbaum DC, van Rhee F, Nabel CS. HHV-8-negative, idiopathic multicentric Castleman disease: novel insights into biology, pathogenesis, and therapy. Blood 2014;123(19):2924–33.
13. Suda T, Katano H, Delsol G, et al. HHV-8 infection status of AIDS-unrelated and AIDS-associated multicentric Castleman's disease. Pathol Int 2001;51(9):671–9.
14. Iwaki N, Fajgenbaum DC, Nabel CS, et al. Clinicopathologic analysis of TAFRO syndrome demonstrates a distinct subtype of HHV-8-negative multicentric Castleman disease. Am J Hematol 2016;91(2):220–6.
15. Fajgenbaum DC, Rosenbach M, van Rhee F, et al. Eruptive cherry hemangiomatosis associated with multicentric Castleman disease: a case report and diagnostic clue. JAMA Dermatol 2013;149(2):204–8.
16. Abdo LA, Morin CP, Collarino RP, et al. First European case of TAFRO syndrome associated with Sjogren disease. Am J Intern Med 2014;2(6):102–5.
17. Jain P, Verstovsek S, Loghavi S, et al. Durable remission with rituximab in a patient with an unusual variant of Castleman's disease with myelofibrosis-TAFRO syndrome. Am J Hematol 2015;90(11):1091–2.
18. Tedesco S, Postacchini L, Manfredi L, et al. Successful treatment of a Caucasian case of multifocal Castleman's disease with TAFRO syndrome with a pathophysiology targeted therapy—a case report. Exp Hematol Oncol 2015;4(1):3.

19. Jouvray M, Terriou L, Meignin V, et al. Pseudo-adult Still's disease, anasarca, thrombotic thrombocytopenic purpura and dysautonomia: an atypical presentation of multicentric Castleman's disease. Discussion of TAFRO syndrome. Rev Med Interne 2016;37(1):53–7 [in French].

20. Jose FF, Kerbauy LN, Perini GF, et al. A life-threatening case of TAFRO syndrome with dramatic response to tocilizumab, rituximab, and pulse steroids: the first case report in Latin America. Medicine 2017;96(13):e6271.

21. Masaki Y, Kawabata H, Takai K, et al. Proposed diagnostic criteria, disease severity classification and treatment strategy for TAFRO syndrome, 2015 version. Int J Hematol 2016;103(6):686–92.

22. Behnia F, Elojeimy S, Matesan M, et al. Potential value of FDG PET-CT in diagnosis and follow-up of TAFRO syndrome. Ann Hematol 2017;96(3):497–500.

23. Kojima M, Nakamura N, Tsukamoto N, et al. Clinical implications of idiopathic multicentric Castleman disease among Japanese: a report of 28 cases. Int J Surg Pathol 2008;16(4):391–8.

24. Kawabata H, Takai K, Kojima M, et al. Castleman-Kojima disease (TAFRO syndrome): a novel systemic inflammatory disease characterized by a constellation of symptoms, namely, thrombocytopenia, ascites (anasarca), microcytic anemia, myelofibrosis, renal dysfunction, and organomegaly: a status report and summary of Fukushima (6 June, 2012) and Nagoya meetings (22 September, 2012). J Clin Exp Hematop 2013;53(1):57–61.

25. Koduri PR, Parvez M, Kaza S, et al. Castleman-Kojima disease in a South Asian adolescent. J Clin Exp Hematop 2014;54(2):163–6.

26. Allegra A, Rotondo F, Russo S, et al. Castleman-Kojima disease (TAFRO syndrome) in a Caucasian patient: a rare case report and review of the literature. Blood Cells Mol Dis 2015;55(3):206–7.

27. Kubokawa I, Yachie A, Hayakawa A, et al. The first report of adolescent TAFRO syndrome, a unique clinicopathologic variant of multicentric Castleman's disease. BMC Pediatr 2014;14:139.

28. Simons M, Apor E, Butera JN, et al. TAFRO syndrome associated with EBV and successful triple therapy treatment: case report and review of the literature. Case Rep Hematol 2016;2016:4703608.

29. Kellam P, Bourboulia D, Dupin N, et al. Characterization of monoclonal antibodies raised against the latent nuclear antigen of human herpesvirus 8. J Virol 1999; 73(6):5149–55.

30. Siegert W, Nerl C, Agthe A, et al. Angioimmunoblastic lymphadenopathy (AILD)-type T-cell lymphoma: prognostic impact of clinical observations and laboratory findings at presentation. The Kiel Lymphoma Study Group. Ann Oncol 1995; 6(7):659–64.

31. Lunning MA, Vose JM. Angioimmunoblastic T-cell lymphoma: the many-faced lymphoma. Blood 2017;129(9):1095–102.

32. Iwaki N, Gion Y, Kondo E, et al. Elevated serum interferon gamma-induced protein 10 kDa is associated with TAFRO syndrome. Sci Rep 2017;7:42316.

33. Liu M, Guo S, Hibbert JM, et al. CXCL10/IP-10 in infectious diseases pathogenesis and potential therapeutic implications. Cytokine Growth Factor Rev 2011; 22(3):121–30.

34. Antonelli A, Ferrari SM, Giuggioli D, et al. Chemokine (C-X-C motif) ligand (CXCL) 10 in autoimmune diseases. Autoimmun Rev 2014;13(3):272–80.

35. Nara M, Komatsuda A, Itoh F, et al. Two cases of thrombocytopenia, anasarca, fever, reticulin fibrosis/renal failure, and organomegaly (TAFRO) syndrome with

high serum procalcitonin levels, including the first case complicated with adrenal hemorrhaging. Intern Med 2017;56(10):1247–52.

36. Assicot M, Gendrel D, Carsin H, et al. High serum procalcitonin concentrations in patients with sepsis and infection. Lancet 1993;341(8844):515–8.

37. Nagai Y, Ando S, Honda N, et al. TAFRO syndrome showing cholangitis on liver biopsy. Rinsho Ketsueki 2016;57(12):2490–5.

38. Takai K, Nikkuni K, Momoi A, et al. Thrombocytopenia with reticulin fibrosis accompanied by fever, anasarca and hepatosplenomegaly: a clinical report of five cases. J Clin Exp Hematop 2013;53(1):63–8.

39. Fajgenbaum DC, Kurzrock R. Siltuximab: a targeted therapy for idiopathic multicentric Castleman disease. Immunotherapy 2016;8(1):17–26.

40. van Rhee F, Wong RS, Munshi N, et al. Siltuximab for multicentric Castleman's disease: a randomised, double-blind, placebo-controlled trial. Lancet Oncol 2014;15(9):966–74.

41. Casper C, Chaturvedi S, Munshi N, et al. Analysis of inflammatory and anemia-related biomarkers in a randomized, double-blind, placebo-controlled study of siltuximab (anti-IL6 monoclonal antibody) in patients with multicentric Castleman disease. Clin Cancer Res 2015;21(19):4294–304.

42. Nishimoto N, Kanakura Y, Aozasa K, et al. Humanized anti-interleukin-6 receptor antibody treatment of multicentric Castleman disease. Blood 2005;106(8): 2627–32.

POEMS Syndrome
Diagnosis and Investigative Work-up

Angela Dispenzieri, MD*, Taxiarchis Kourelis, MD, Francis Buadi, MD

KEYWORDS

- Chronic inflammatory polyradiculoneuropathy • Plasma cell disorder
- Castleman disease • Paraneoplastic

KEY POINTS

- Plasma cell disorder and length-dependent peripheral neuropathy should suggest POEMS as a diagnosis.
- The presence of thrombocytosis should further heighten the index of suspicion.
- Vascular endothelial growth factor, bone marrow biopsy, and computed tomography imaging of bones are key in making the diagnosis.
- Early diagnosis and thorough baseline evaluation are important.

INTRODUCTION

The diagnosis of POEMS (polyneuropathy, organomegaly, endocrinopathy, M protein, skin changes) syndrome is made based on a composite of clinical and laboratory features (**Table 1**).[1] It is a rare disorder with a reported prevalence of approximately 0.3 per 100,000.[2] The peak incidence of the POEMS syndrome is in the fifth and sixth decades of life, unlike multiple myeloma (MM), which has a peak incidence in the seventh and eighth decades. The constellation of neuropathy and any of the following should elicit an in-depth search for POEMS syndrome: monoclonal protein (especially lambda light chain), thrombocytosis, anasarca, or papilledema. Any patient who carries a diagnosis of chronic inflammatory demyelinating polyneuropathy (CIDP) that is not responding to standard CIDP therapy should be considered as possibly having POEMS syndrome, and additional testing should be done to rule in or rule out the diagnosis of POEMS syndrome. A good history and physical examination followed by appropriate testing, most notably radiographic assessment of bones,[3–5] measurement of vascular endothelial growth factor (VEGF),[6–10] and careful analysis of a bone marrow biopsy[11] can differentiate this syndrome from other conditions like CIDP, monoclonal gammopathy of undetermined significance (MGUS), neuropathy, and

Division of Hematology, Department of Medicine, Medicine, Mayo Clinic, 200 First Street Southwest, Rochester, MN 55905, USA
* Corresponding author.
E-mail address: Dispenzieri.angela@mayo.edu

Hematol Oncol Clin N Am 32 (2018) 119–139
https://doi.org/10.1016/j.hoc.2017.09.010
0889-8588/18/© 2017 Elsevier Inc. All rights reserved.

Table 1 Criteria for the diagnosis of POEMS syndrome[a]	
Mandatory major criteria	1. Polyneuropathy (typically demyelinating) 2. Monoclonal plasma cell proliferative disorder (almost always lambda)
Other major criteria (1 required)	3. Castleman disease[a] 4. Sclerotic bone lesions 5. Increased levels of vascular endothelial growth factor
Minor criteria	6. Organomegaly (splenomegaly, hepatomegaly, or lymphadenopathy) 7. Extravascular volume overload (edema, pleural effusion, or ascites) 8. Endocrinopathy (adrenal, thyroid,[b] pituitary, gonadal, parathyroid, pancreatic[b]) 9. Skin changes (hyperpigmentation, hypertrichosis, glomeruloid hemangiomata, plethora, acrocyanosis, flushing, white nails) 10. Papilledema 11. Thrombocytosis/polycythemia[c]
Other symptoms and signs	Clubbing, weight loss, hyperhidrosis, pulmonary hypertension/restrictive lung disease, thrombotic diatheses, diarrhea, low vitamin B_{12} values

The diagnosis of POEMS syndrome is confirmed when both of the mandatory major criteria, 1 of the 3 other major criteria, and 1 of the 6 minor criteria are present.

[a] There is a Castleman disease variant of POEMS syndrome that occurs without evidence of a clonal plasma cell disorder that is not accounted for in this table. This entity should be considered separately.

[b] Because of the high prevalence of diabetes mellitus and thyroid abnormalities, this diagnosis alone is not sufficient to meet this minor criterion.

[c] Approximately 50% of patients have bone marrow changes that distinguish it from a typical monoclonal gammopathy of undetermined significance or myeloma bone marrow. Anemia and/or thrombocytopenia are distinctively unusual in this syndrome unless Castleman disease is present.

From Dispenzieri A. POEMS syndrome: update on diagnosis, risk-stratification, and management. Am J Hematol 2015;90(10):953; with permission.

immunoglobulin light chain amyloid neuropathy. As discussed later, there is a Castleman variant of POEMS syndrome that does not have a clonal plasma cell proliferative disorder underlying but has many of the other paraneoplastic features.[12]

HISTORY

Scheinker's[13] autopsy case in 1938 was the first report of what is now called POEMS syndrome.[13–16] His patient was a 39-year-old man with a solitary plasmacytoma, sensorimotor polyneuropathy, and localized patches of thickened and deeply pigmented skin on the chest.[13,17] The complexity of the interaction of plasma cell dyscrasia and peripheral neuropathy became increasingly evident in 1956 with Crow's[18] description of 2 patients with osteosclerotic plasmacytomas with neuropathy, and other striking features, which included clubbing, skin pigmentation, dusky discoloration of skin, white fingernails, mild lymphadenopathy, and ankle edema.[18] As many as 50% of patients with osteosclerotic myeloma were noted to have peripheral neuropathy,[17,19,20] in contrast with 1% to 8% of patients with multiple myeloma.[21,22] Other investigators reported patients with osteosclerotic myeloma and peripheral neuropathy with organomegaly, skin changes, endocrinopathy, edema, hypertrichosis, gynecomastia, and ascites.[17,23–28] A syndrome distinct from multiple myeloma–associated neuropathy began to be recognized. In Iwashita and colleagues'[17] 1977 review of the literature, the 30 patients with osteosclerotic myeloma and peripheral neuropathy, compared with the 29 patients without peripheral neuropathy, more commonly had hyperpigmentation, edema, skin thickening, hepatomegaly, hypertrichosis, and clubbing.

In 1980, Bardwick and colleagues[16] described 2 patients and coined the acronym POEMS. In 1981, Kelly and colleagues[29] reported on 16 cases seen at Mayo, and in 1983[30] and 1984[14] 2 large series of cases collected from Japan were reported supporting the existence of a distinct pathologic entity. Over the years, additional large series have been reported.[14,30–33] Estimated frequencies of findings are shown in **Table 2**. The variability between series is most likely a function of retrospective reporting (ie, if a physician does not order a test or chart a finding, it will not be captured) and local practices, and promptness of diagnosis, rather than ethnic differences.

PATHOPHYSIOLOGY

The real mechanism involved in the pathogenesis of POEMS syndrome is still unknown, but cytokines may play a major role. Plasma and serum levels of VEGF are markedly increased in patients with POEMS[10,34–36] and correlate with the activity of the disease.[6,7,10,35] The principal isoform of VEGF expressed is VEGF165.[6] VEGF levels are independent of M-protein size.[6] Increased VEGF has been found in ascitic fluid[37] and the cerebrospinal fluid.[7] In a recent study, Wang and colleagues[38] showed that the bone marrow plasma cells of patients with POEMS syndrome had higher levels of VEGF messenger RNA expression than did their CD138-negative cells. A remarkable observation was that polyclonal plasma cells and clonal plasma cells had equally high levels of intracellular VEGF, although monoclonal PCs had higher levels of intracellular interleukin (IL)-6 expression. IL-1β, tumor necrosis factor alpha (TNF-α), and IL-6 levels are often also increased. IL-12 has also been shown to correlate with disease activity.[39] Exactly how these cytokines effect the changes observed in patients is unclear.

In an animal model, VEGF increased the microvascular permeability inducing endoneurial edema.[40,41] The investigators postulate that this increased permeability could allow serum components toxic to nerves, like complement and thrombin, to induce further damage. Scarlato and colleagues[7] proposed that the mechanism of peripheral neuropathy in POEMS syndrome is caused by endothelial injury, indirectly or directly caused by an abnormal activation of endothelial cells by VEGF, which is overexpressed in the nerves of patients with POEMS syndrome. According to these investigators, there may be hypertrophy and proliferation of endothelial cells with a secondary microangiopathy that fuels the destructive feedback loop of reduced oxygen supply, expression of hypoxia-inducible factor 1a, with a secondary increase in local VEGF expression. In another study of human nerve biopsies of patients with POEMS, more than 50% of endoneurial blood vessels had narrowed or closed lumina with thick basement membranes, strong polyclonal immunoglobulin staining in the endoneurium (consistent with blood-nerve barrier opening), and thrombin-antithrombin complexes immunohistochemically.[42]

PERIPHERAL NEUROPATHY

The neuropathy is the dominant characteristic of the syndrome. The quality and extent of the neuropathy, which is peripheral, ascending, symmetric, and affecting both

Table 2
Summary of frequencies of POEMS syndrome findings based on large retrospective series

Characteristic	Affected (%)[a]
Polyneuropathy	100
Organomegaly	45–85
Hepatomegaly	24–78
Splenomegaly	22–70
Lymphadenopathy	26–74
Castleman disease	11–25
Endocrinopathy	67–84
Gonadal axis abnormality	55–89
Adrenal axis abnormality	16–33
Increased prolactin value	5–20
Gynecomastia or galactorrhea	12–18
Diabetes mellitus	3–36
Hypothyroidism	9–67
Monoclonal plasma cell dyscrasia[b]	100
M protein on serum protein electrophoresis	24–54
Skin changes	68–89
Hyperpigmentation	46–93
Acrocyanosis and plethora	19
Hemangioma/telangiectasia	9–35
Hypertrichosis	26–74
Thickening	5–43
Papilledema	29–64
Extravascular volume overload	29–87
Peripheral edema	24–89
Ascites	7–54
Pleural effusion	3–43
Pericardial effusion	1–64
Bone lesions	27–97
Thrombocytosis	54–88
Polycythemia	12–19
Clubbing	5–49
Decreased carbon monoxide diffusion in the lung	>15
Pulmonary hypertension	36
Weight loss >4.5 kg (10 lb)	37
Fatigue	31

[a] Percentages are based on the total number of patients in the series.
[b] In both the Takasuki[30] and Nakanishi[14] series, only 75% of patients had a documented plasma cell disorder, which defies the current definition for POEMS syndrome. Because these are among the earliest series describing the syndrome, they are included.
From Dispenzieri A. POEMS syndrome: update on diagnosis, risk-stratification, and management. Am J Hematol 2015;90(10):955; with permission.

sensation and motor function, should be elicited.[29] It starts as a sensory neuropathy and motor symptoms typically dominate over time. In our experience, pain may be a dominant feature in about 10% to 15% of patients, and in one report as many as

76% of patients had hyperesthesia.[2,43] Patients are areflexic and typically have a step-page gait and a positive Romberg sign.

Nerve conduction studies in patients with POEMS syndrome show slowing of nerve conduction that is more predominant in the intermediate than distal nerve segments compared with CIDP, and there is more severe attenuation of compound muscle action potentials in the lower than upper limbs.[2,44–47] In contrast with CIDP, conduction block is rare.[2,45,47] The conduction findings could suggest that demyelination is predominant in the nerve trunk rather than the distal nerve terminals and axonal loss is predominant in the lower limb nerves.[2] Axonal loss is greater in POEMS syndrome than it is in CIDP.[47] The nerve biopsy shows typical features of uncompacted myelin lamellae. At ultrastructural examination there are no features of macrophage-associated demyelination, which are seen in some cases of chronic inflammatory demyelinating polyneuropathy.[48–51] In one report, the presence of hyperalgesia was closely related to a reduction in the myelinated, but not unmyelinated, fiber population.[52] In another study, ultrastuctural analysis of POEMS nerves revealed endothelial cytoplasmic enlargement, opening of the tight junctions between endothelial cells, and presence of many pinocytic vesicles adjacent to the cell membranes, all consistent with an alteration of the permeability of endoneurial vessels.[7]

MONOCLONAL PLASMA CELL DISORDER AND HEMATOLOGIC FINDINGS

The size of the M protein on electrophoresis is small (median, 1.1 g/dL) and is rarely more than 3.0 g/dL. The M protein is usually immunoglobulin (Ig) G or IgA and almost always of the lambda type.[30,31] Laboratory findings are notable for an absence of cytopenias. Nearly half of patients have thrombocytosis or erythrocytosis.[31] In the series of Li and colleagues,[32] 26% of patients had anemia, which the investigators attributed to impaired renal function. Their series was enriched with Castleman disease cases (25%), which may have also contributed to this unprecedentedly high rate of anemia.

Bone marrow usually contains less than 5% plasma cells, and, when clonal cells are found, they are almost always monoclonal lambda. Little is known about the plasma cells in POEMS syndrome except that more than 95% of the time they are lambda light chain restricted with restricted immunoglobulin light chain variable gene usage (IGLV1).[53–55] Translocations and deletion of chromosome 13 have been described, but hyperdiploidy is not seen.[56,57]

The bone marrow biopsy reveals megakaryocyte hyperplasia and megakaryocyte clustering in 54% and 93% of cases, respectively.[11] These megakaryocyte findings are reminiscent of a myeloproliferative disorder, but *JAK2*V617F mutation is uniformly absent. One-third of patients do not have clonal plasma cells on their iliac crest biopsies. These are the patients who present with a solitary or multiple solitary plasmacytomas. The other two-thirds of patients have clonal plasma cells in their bone marrows, and 91% of these cases are clonal lambda. Immunohistochemical staining is more sensitive than is 6-color flow because the former provides information on bone marrow architecture, which is key in making the diagnosis in nearly half of cases. In our study of 67 pretreatment bone marrows biopsies from patients with POEMS syndrome, lymphoid aggregates were found in 49% of cases. Of these, there was plasma cell rimming in all but 1, and in 75% and 4% the rimming was clonal lambda and kappa, respectively. This finding was not seen in bone marrows from normal controls or from patients with MGUS, multiple myeloma, or amyloidosis. Overall, only 8 out of 67 (12%) POEMS cases had normal iliac crest bone marrow biopsies; that is, no detectable clonal plasma cells, no plasma cell–rimmed lymphoid aggregates, and no megakaryocyte hyperplasia.

BONE LESIONS

Osteosclerotic lesions occur in approximately 95% of patients, and can be confused with benign bone islands, aneurysmal bone cysts, nonossifying fibromas, and fibrous dysplasia.[14,31,58,59] Some lesions are densely sclerotic, whereas others are lytic with a sclerotic rim, whereas still others have a mixed soap-bubble appearance (**Fig. 1**). Bone windows of computed tomography (CT) body images are often very informative, even more so than fluorodeoxyglucose (FDG) uptake, which can be variable.[4,5] FDG uptake occurs in those lesions that have a lytic component.[60] The advantage of whole-body CT (even low dose, similar to what is quickly becoming the standard in multiple myeloma) is that other features of the disease are also seen: effusions, ascites, adenopathy, and hepatosplenomegaly.

EXTRAVASCULAR VOLUME OVERLOAD

Extravascular fluid overload most commonly manifests as peripheral edema, but pleural effusion, ascites, and pericardial effusions are also common. The composition of the ascites was studied in 42 patients with POEMS syndrome. The ascitic fluid had low serum ascites albumin gradients consistent with an exudative rather than a portal hypertension process in 74% of cases.[61]

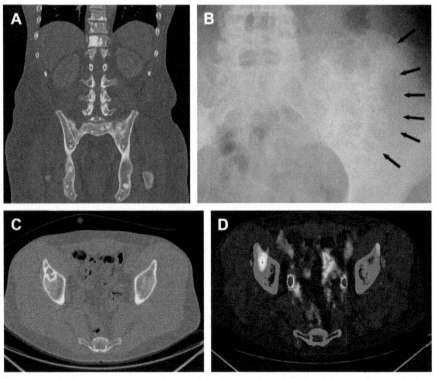

Fig. 1. Bone lesions in POEMS syndrome. (*A*) Diffuse sclerotic lesions seen on bone windows of computed tomography scan. (*B*) Mixed lytic and sclerotic lesion, soap-bubble lesion. (*C*) Lytic lesion with sclerotic rim right ischium. (*D*) Fluorodeoxyglucose avidity of lesion seen in **Fig. 1C**.

VASCULAR ENDOTHELIAL GROWTH FACTOR AND OTHER CYTOKINES

Plasma and serum levels of VEGF are markedly increased in patients with POEMS[10,34–36] and correlate with the activity of the disease.[6,7,10,35] The principal isoform of VEGF expressed is VEGF165.[6] VEGF levels are independent of M-protein size.[6] Increased VEGF has been found in ascitic fluid[37] and the cerebrospinal fluid.[7] IL-1β, TNF-α, and IL-6 levels are often also increased. Serum VEGF levels are 10 to 50 times higher than plasma levels of VEGF.[62] In patients with POEMS, VEGF is found in both plasma cells[63,64] and platelets.[36] The higher level observed in serum is attributable to the release of VEGF from platelets in vitro during serum processing. Because plasma is a product of an anticoagulated sample, there is less platelet activation and therefore less platelet VEGF contributing to the plasma measurement than the serum sample. Tokashiki and colleagues[62] suggest that serum VEGF is the better test because it reflects the VEGF contribution from both the serous and platelet compartments. However, the counterargument is that the amount of VEGF release by platelets may vary because of collection and processing technique, making serum measurements of VEGF less reliable. The authors have shown that a plasma VEGF level of 200 pg/mL had a specificity of 95% with a sensitivity of 68% in support of a diagnosis of POEMS syndrome. Other diseases with high VEGF levels include connective tissue disease and vasculitis.[10] Others investigators have shown that a serum level of 1920 pg/mL is diagnostic of POEMS with a specificity of 98% and a sensitivity of 73%.[65]

ORGANOMEGALY

As many as three-quarters of patients have organomegaly, but other series suggest that it occurs in only one-quarter of patients.[14,30–33,66] Any or all of liver, spleen, and lymph nodes can be enlarged. Between 11% and 30% of patients with POEMS who have a documented clonal plasma cell disorder also have documented Castleman disease or Castleman-like histology.[14,16,31–33] In 30 patients with POEMS syndrome, 19 of 32 biopsied lymph nodes showed angiofollicular hyperplasia typical of Castleman disease.[14] In another series, 25 of 43 biopsied lymph nodes were diagnostic of Castleman disease and 84% of these had hyaline vascular type.[32]

Castleman disease (or angiofollicular lymph node hyperplasia) is a rare lymphoproliferative disorder that has many presentations, ranging from an asymptomatic unifocal mass to multifocal masses with a multitude of symptoms. The symptoms can range from simple B symptoms to various autoimmune phenomena to a frank POEMS syndrome.[14,31,33,67–100]

ENDOCRINOPATHY

Endocrinopathy is a central but poorly understood feature of POEMS. In one large series,[66] approximately 84% of patients had a recognized endocrinopathy, with hypogonadism as the most common endocrine abnormality, followed by thyroid abnormalities, glucose metabolism abnormalities, and by adrenal insufficiency. Most patients have evidence of multiple endocrinopathies in the 4 major endocrine axes (gonadal, thyroid, glucose, and adrenal).

SKIN FINDINGS

A whole-skin examination should be performed looking for hyperpigmentation, a recent outcropping of hemangioma, hypertrichosis, dependent rubor and acrocyanosis, lipodystrophy, white nails, sclerodermoid changes, facial atrophy, flushing, or clubbing.[30,32,33,101–105] Rarely calciphylaxis is also seen.[106,107] In our experience, fingernail clubbing is seen in about 4% of cases, but others have reported rates as high as 49%.[14,108]

The histologic findings of the dermis have been reported to range from nonspecific to glomeruloid hemangiomata to vascular abnormalities in apparently normal dermis.[109–111] Biopsies of normal-appearing skin showed an extremely complex subpapillary vascular network with largely dilated and frequently anastomotic vessels.[112] Capillary loops appeared more complex than normal, and most of them were probably clotted.

PAPILLEDEMA

Papilledema is present in at least one-third of patients. Of the 33 patients at our institution referred for a formal ophthalmologic examination during a 10-year period, 67% had ocular signs and symptoms, the most common of which was papilledema in 52% of those examined.[113] The most common ocular symptoms reported were blurred vision in 15, diplopia in 5, and ocular pain in 3. In another series of 94 patients, papilledema, which was found in approximately 50% of patients, was an adverse prognostic feature for overall survival.[114]

RESPIRATORY FINDINGS

The pulmonary manifestations are protean, including pulmonary hypertension, restrictive lung disease, impaired neuromuscular respiratory function, and impaired diffusion capacity of carbon monoxide, but these improve with effective therapy (**Fig. 2**).[108,115] Respiratory complaints are usually limited given patients' neurologic status impairing their ability to induce cardiovascular challenges. In a series of 137 patients with POEMS syndrome seen at our institution between 1975 and 2003, at presentation the frequencies with which patients reported dyspnea, chest pain, cough, and orthopnea were 20%, 10%, 8%, and 7%, respectively.[108] Nearly 25% had significant chest roentgenogram abnormalities.

Pulmonary hypertension has been reported to occur in approximately 25% of patients with POEMS syndrome.[115,116] It is more likely to occur in patients with extravascular overload. Whether the digital clubbing seen in POEMS is a reflection of underlying pulmonary hypertension and/or parenchymal disease is yet to be determined. Impaired carbon monoxide diffusion in the lung has been shown to be an adverse prognostic factor in another series.[114]

RENAL FINDINGS

Serum creatinine levels are normal in most patients, but serum cystatin C level, which is a surrogate marker for renal function, is high in 71% of patients.[117] In our experience, at presentation, fewer than 10% of patients have proteinuria exceeding 0.5 g/24 h, and only 6% have a serum creatinine level greater than or equal to 1.5 mg/dL. Four percent of patients developed renal failure as a preterminal event.[31] In another series from China, 37% of patients had a creatinine clearance (CrCl) of less than 60 mL/min/m^2, and 9% had a CrCl of less than 30 mL/min/m^2 and 15% had microhematuria.[32] The estimate of CrCl level less than 60 mL/min/m^2 has recently been revised to 22% of patients by the same group from China.[118] In our experience, renal disease is more likely to occur in patients who have coexisting Castleman disease. In POEMS syndrome, the renal histologic findings are diverse with membranoproliferative features and evidence of endothelial injury being most common.[119] On both light and electron microscopy, mesangial expansion, narrowing of capillary lumina,

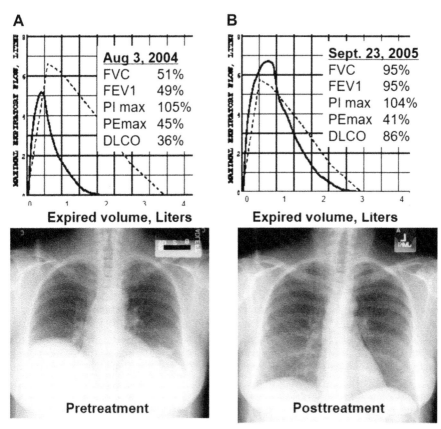

Fig. 2. Pulmonary findings before and after therapy. (*A*) Pretreatment pulmonary function tests and chest radiograph. (*B*) Posttreatment pulmonary function tests and chest radiograph.

basement membrane thickening, subendothelial deposits, widening of the subendothelial space, swelling and vacuolization of endothelial cells, and mesangiolysis predominate.[120–126] Standard immunofluorescence is negative,[121,127] which differentiates it from primary membranoproliferative glomerulitis.[119] Rarely, infiltration by plasma cells nests or Castleman-like lymphoma can be seen.[126]

THROMBOSIS

Patients are at increased risk for arterial and/or venous thromboses during their course, with nearly 20% of patients experiencing one of these complications.[128,129] Lesprit and colleagues[128] observed 4 out of 20 patients to have arterial occlusion. In the Mayo series, there were 18 patients who had serious events such as stroke, myocardial infarction, and Budd-Chiari syndrome.[31] Affected vessels include carotid, iliac, celiac, subclavian, mesenteric, and femoral.[130–133] Ten percent of patients presented with a cerebrovascular event, most commonly embolic or vessel dissection and stenosis.[134] The POEMS-associated strokes tend to be end-artery border-zone infarctions.[133] The median time between peripheral neuropathy symptom onset and the cerebrovascular event was 23 months (range, 0.5–64 months). Risk factors for cerebral events included thrombocytosis and bone marrow plasmacytosis. Aberrations in the coagulation cascade have been implicated in POEMS syndrome.[42] In one report, levels of circulating coagulation factors like fibrinopeptide A and thrombin-antithrombin complex increased during the active phase of illness, but other factors relating to fibrinolysis, plasminogen, a2-plasmin inhibitor–plasmin complex, and fibrin degradation products did not increase.

OTHER LABORATORY FINDINGS

Levels of serum erythropoietin are low and are inversely correlated with VEGF levels.[7] Bence Jones proteinuria is uncommon. Protein levels in the cerebrospinal fluid are increased in virtually all patients. Plasma cells are not present in the cerebrospinal fluid, but increased levels of IL-6 receptor [135] and VEGF[7] have been described. Wang and colleagues[65] identified N-terminal propeptide of type I collagen as a novel marker for the diagnosis of patients with POEMS. They found that the best cutoff of N-terminal propeptide of type I collagen to diagnosis POEMS syndrome is 70 ng/mL, with a specificity of 91.5% and a sensitivity of 80%.

DIFFERENTIAL DIAGNOSIS

The differential diagnosis of POEMS is vast. The most common differential diagnoses lie in the realm of peripheral neuropathies, like CIDP. Rarely, a patient is diagnosed as having Guillain-Barré. If the monoclonal protein is recognized, it can mistakenly be diagnosed as MGUS, smoldering myeloma, solitary plasmacytoma, or overt myeloma. If a patient with POEMS syndrome is incorrectly deemed to have an MGUS or smoldering multiple myeloma, then no treatment directed at the clone will be recommended, existing symptoms will worsen, and the patient will accumulate additional elements of the paraneoplastic syndrome. If the patient is incorrectly diagnosed with MM or plasmacytoma, and standard therapies for these disorders are administered, there will likely be increased treatment-related morbidity and inadequate supportive care.

Osteosclerotic lesions occur in approximately 95% of patients and can be confused with benign bone islands, aneurysmal bone cysts, nonossifying fibromas, and fibrous dysplasia. Some lesions are densely sclerotic, whereas others are lytic with a sclerotic rim, whereas still others have a mixed soap-bubble appearance (see **Fig. 1**). Bone windows of CT body images are often very informative. FDG avidity is variable.

High VEGF levels can be seen in connective tissue diseases and in Castleman disease. Several published cases of so-called interesting features associated with Castleman disease are likely cases of POEMS syndrome.[136–139] In contrast with the osteosclerotic myeloma variant of POEMS in which VEGF is the most consistently increased cytokine, in Castleman disease IL-6 is the dominant aberrantly overexpressed cytokine. Multicentric Castleman disease with and without peripheral neuropathy tends to be different; it has even been proposed that the presence or absence of peripheral neuropathy should be part of the multicentric Castleman disease classification system.[140] Those patients with peripheral neuropathy are more likely to have edema and impaired peripheral circulation,[137,141–146] and they are also more likely to have a monoclonal lambda protein in their serum and/or urine.[147]

The neuropathy in patients with Castleman disease tends to be more subtle than that of patients with POEMS with osteosclerotic myeloma and is more often sensory. However, at its worst, it is a mixture of demyelination and axonal degeneration with normal myelin spacing on electron microscopy,[145] and abnormal capillary proliferation, similar to what is seen in the affected lymph nodes, has been described.[145]

Table 3
Recommended minimum testing

Test	Baseline	Every 3–6 mo	Yearly
Neurologic			
Detailed neurologic history (numbness, pain, weakness, balance, orthostasis) and examination (including funduscopic examination)	X	X[a]	X
Electrophysiologic study (nerve conduction studies)	X	X[a]	X
Sural nerve biopsy	X[d]	—	—
Organomegaly/Lymphadenopathy/Extravascular Volume Overload			
Physical examination and CT scan documenting lymphadenopathy, organomegaly, ascites, pleural effusions, and edema	X	X[b]	X[b]
Endocrinopathy			
History regarding menstrual and sexual function	X	X	X
Testosterone, estradiol, fasting glucose, glycosylated hemoglobin, thyroid-stimulating hormone, parathyroid hormone, prolactin, serum cortisol, luteinizing hormone	X	X[b]	X[b]
Follicle-stimulating hormone, adrenocorticotropin hormone, Cortrosyn stimulation test	X[d]	X[b]	X[b]
Hematologic			
Serum protein electrophoresis and immunofixation	X	X	X
Affected quantitative immunoglobulin	X	X[d]	X
Complete blood count (hemoglobin, platelets)	X	X	X
24-h urine total protein, electrophoresis, and immunofixation	X	—	X
Vascular endothelial growth factor	X	X	X
Bone marrow aspirate and biopsy (test for kappa/lambda by immunohistochemistry)	X	X[c]	—
Skin			
History and physical with attention to skin pigment, thickening, and texture; body hair quantity and texture; color of distal extremities; and development of cherry angiomata	X	X	X
Sclerotic Bone Lesions			
CT body bone windows and/or PET/CT	X	—	X[d]
Pulmonary Function			
Pulmonary function tests	X	X[b]	X[b]
Echocardiography to assess right ventricular systolic and pulmonary artery pressures	X	X[b]	X[b]

[a] At 6 months and then yearly.
[b] Only if affected.
[c] Only to document complete response.
[d] As clinically indicated.
Modified from Dispenzieri A. POEMS syndrome: update on diagnosis, risk-stratification, and management. Am J Hematol 2015;90(10):954; with permission.

Patients with Castleman disease often have a brisk polyclonal hypergammaglobuline-mia. Only those with peripheral neuropathy and a plasma cell clone should be classified as having standard POEMS syndrome. Without both of these characteristics, patients can be classified as having Castleman disease variant of POEMS if they have other POEMS features.

TESTING GUIDELINES

To screen for POEMS in a patient with a monoclonal gammopathy and a length-dependent peripheral neuropathy (especially if it is demyelinating), clinicians should perform either low-resolution CT body with bone windows or PET/CT along with a VEGF level. If neither of these is consistent with the diagnosis, the patient either does not have POEMS syndrome or perhaps has very early disease.

Once a diagnosis is made, patients with POEMS syndrome should be thoroughly evaluated to define a baseline that can be used for future assessments (**Table 3**). Once patients begin therapy, monthly testing of the monoclonal protein and VEGF levels is most typical. With completion of therapy, VEGF and monoclonal protein testing can be done less frequently: initially every 3 months, and then every 3 to 6 months. Imaging and neurology testing are recommended initially every 6 months followed by annually. For those patients in complete hematologic response and complete VEGF and PET scan response, imaging can be done less frequently.

SUMMARY POINTS

POEMS is a complex but fascinating syndrome that shares elements with other diseases, most notably other plasma cell dyscrasias and Castleman disease. Unraveling the elements of this paraneoplastic syndrome has the potential to provide insight into several other disorders. Major hints for the diagnosis are a lambda restricted plasma cell disorder and a length-dependent peripheral neuropathy. Thrombocytosis can also be a clue in that it is present in 54% of patients with POEMS.[148–173] Immunohistochemistry of the bone marrow can also be pathognomonic for a diagnosis.

REFERENCES

1. Dispenzieri A. POEMS syndrome: update on diagnosis, risk-stratification, and management. Am J Hematol 2015;90(10):951–62.
2. Nasu S, Misawa S, Sekiguchi Y, et al. Different neurological and physiological profiles in POEMS syndrome and chronic inflammatory demyelinating polyneuropathy. J Neurol Neurosurg Psychiatry 2012;83(5):476–9.
3. Alberti MA, Martinez-Yelamos S, Fernandez A, et al. 18F-FDG PET/CT in the evaluation of POEMS syndrome. Eur J Radiol 2010;76(2):180–2.
4. Glazebrook K, Guerra Bonilla FL, Johnson A, et al. Computed tomography assessment of bone lesions in patients with POEMS syndrome. Eur Radiol 2015;25(2):497–504.
5. Shi X, Hu S, Luo X, et al. CT characteristics in 24 patients with POEMS syndrome. Acta Radiol 2016;57(1):51–7.
6. Watanabe O, Maruyama I, Arimura K, et al. Overproduction of vascular endothelial growth factor/vascular permeability factor is causative in Crow-Fukase (POEMS) syndrome. Muscle Nerve 1998;21(11):1390–7.
7. Scarlato M, Previtali SC, Carpo M, et al. Polyneuropathy in POEMS syndrome: role of angiogenic factors in the pathogenesis. Brain 2005;128(Pt 8):1911–20.
8. Nobile-Orazio E, Terenghi F, Giannotta C, et al. Serum VEGF levels in POEMS syndrome and in immune-mediated neuropathies. Neurology 2009;72(11):1024–6.

9. Briani C, Fabrizi GM, Ruggero S, et al. Vascular endothelial growth factor helps differentiate neuropathies in rare plasma cell dyscrasias. Muscle Nerve 2010; 43(2):164–7.
10. D'Souza A, Hayman SR, Buadi F, et al. The utility of plasma vascular endothelial growth factor levels in the diagnosis and follow-up of patients with POEMS syndrome. Blood 2011;118(17):4663–5.
11. Dao LN, Hanson CA, Dispenzieri A, et al. Bone marrow histopathology in POEMS syndrome: a distinctive combination of plasma cell, lymphoid and myeloid findings in 87 patients. Blood 2011;117(24):6438–44.
12. Dispenzieri A. Castleman disease. Cancer Treat Res 2008;142:293–330.
13. Scheinker L. Myelom und Nervensystem: uber eine bisher nicht beschrieben mit eigentumlichen Hautveranderungen einhergehende Polyneuritis bei einem plamazellularen Myelom des Sternums. Dtsch Z Nervenheilkd 1938;147:247–73.
14. Nakanishi T, Sobue I, Toyokura Y, et al. The Crow-Fukase syndrome: a study of 102 cases in Japan. Neurology 1984;34(6):712–20.
15. Driedger H, Pruzanski W. Plasma cell neoplasia with peripheral polyneuropathy. A study of five cases and a review of the literature. Medicine 1980;59(4):301–10.
16. Bardwick PA, Zvaifler NJ, Gill GN, et al. Plasma cell dyscrasia with polyneuropathy, organomegaly, endocrinopathy, M protein, and skin changes: the POEMS syndrome. Report on two cases and a review of the literature. Medicine 1980; 59(4):311–22.
17. Iwashita H, Ohnishi A, Asada M, et al. Polyneuropathy, skin hyperpigmentation, edema, and hypertrichosis in localized osteosclerotic myeloma. Neurology 1977;27(7):675–81.
18. Crow RS. Peripheral neuritis in myelomatosis. Br Med J 1956;2(4996):802–4.
19. Driedger H, Pruzanski W. Plasma cell neoplasia with osteosclerotic lesions. A study of five cases and a review of the literature. Arch Intern Med 1979; 139(8):892–6.
20. Mangalik A, Veliath AJ. Osteosclerotic myeloma and peripheral neuropathy. A case report. Cancer 1971;28(4):1040–5.
21. Evison G, Evans KT. Sclerotic bone deposits in multiple myeloma [letter]. Br J Radiol 1983;56(662):145.
22. Reitan JB, Pape E, Fossa SD, et al. Osteosclerotic myeloma with polyneuropathy. Acta Med Scand 1980;208(1–2):137–44.
23. Morley JB, Schwieger AC. The relation between chronic polyneuropathy and osteosclerotic myeloma. J Neurol Neurosurg Psychiatry 1967;30(5):432–42.
24. Mayo CM, Daniels A, Barron KD. Polyneuropathy in the osteosclerotic form of multiple myeloma. Trans Am Neurol Assoc 1968;93:240–2.
25. Shimpo S, Nishitani H, Tsunermura T. Solitary plasmacytoma with polyneuritis and endocrine disturbance. Nihon Rinsho 1968;26:2444–56 [in Japanese].
26. Imawari M, Akatsuka N, Ishibashi M, et al. Syndrome of plasma cell dyscrasia, polyneuropathy, and endocrine disturbances. Report of a case. Ann Intern Med 1974;81(4):490–3.
27. Amiel J, Machover D, Droz J. Plasma cell dyscrasia with arteriopathy, polyneuropathy, and endocrine syndrome. A Japanese disease in an Italian patient. Ann Med Interne (Paris) 1975;126(11):745–9 [in French].
28. Waldenstrom JG, Adner A, Gydell K, et al. Osteosclerotic "plasmocytoma" with polyneuropathy, hypertrichosis and diabetes. Acta Med Scand 1978;203(4): 297–303.
29. Kelly JJ Jr, Kyle RA, Miles JM, et al. Osteosclerotic myeloma and peripheral neuropathy. Neurology 1983;33(2):202–10.

30. Takatsuki K, Sanada I. Plasma cell dyscrasia with polyneuropathy and endo-crine disorder: clinical and laboratory features of 109 reported cases. Jpn J Clin Oncol 1983;13(3):543–55.
31. Dispenzieri A, Kyle RA, Lacy MQ, et al. POEMS syndrome: definitions and long-term outcome. Blood 2003;101(7):2496–506.
32. Li J, Zhou DB, Huang Z, et al. Clinical characteristics and long-term outcome of patients with POEMS syndrome in China. Ann Hematol 2011;90(7):819–26.
33. Soubrier MJ, Dubost JJ, Sauvezie BJ. POEMS syndrome: a study of 25 cases and a review of the literature. French Study Group on POEMS Syndrome. Am J Med 1994;97(6):543–53.
34. Watanabe O, Arimura K, Kitajima I, et al. Greatly raised vascular endothelial growth factor (VEGF) in POEMS syndrome [letter]. Lancet 1996;347(9002):702.
35. Soubrier M, Dubost JJ, Serre AF, et al. Growth factors in POEMS syndrome: ev-idence for a marked increase in circulating vascular endothelial growth factor. Arthritis Rheum 1997;40(4):786–7.
36. Hashiguchi T, Arimura K, Matsumuro K, et al. Highly concentrated vascular endothelial growth factor in platelets in Crow-Fukase syndrome. Muscle Nerve 2000;23(7):1051–6.
37. Loeb JM, Hauger PH, Carney JD, et al. Refractory ascites due to POEMS syn-drome. Gastroenterology 1989;96(1):247–9.
38. Wang C, Huang XF, Cai QQ, et al. Remarkable expression of vascular endothe-lial growth factor in bone marrow plasma cells of patients with POEMS syn-drome. Leuk Res 2016;50:78–84.
39. Kanai K, Sawai S, Sogawa K, et al. Markedly upregulated serum interleukin-12 as a novel biomarker in POEMS syndrome. Neurology 2012;79(6):575–82.
40. Arimura K. Increased vascular endothelial growth factor (VEGF) is causative in Crow-Fukase syndrome. Rinsho Shinkeigaku 1999;39(1):84–5 [in Japanese].
41. Soubrier M, Sauron C, Souweine B, et al. Growth factors and proinflammatory cytokines in the renal involvement of POEMS syndrome. Am J Kidney Dis 1999;34(4):633–8.
42. Saida K, Kawakami H, Ohta M, et al. Coagulation and vascular abnormalities in Crow-Fukase syndrome. Muscle Nerve 1997;20(4):486–92.
43. Koike H, Iijima M, Mori K, et al. Neuropathic pain correlates with myelinated fibre loss and cytokine profile in POEMS syndrome. J Neurol Neurosurg Psychiatry 2008;79(10):1171–9.
44. Kelly JJ Jr. The electrodiagnostic findings in peripheral neuropathy associated with monoclonal gammopathy. Muscle Nerve 1983;6(7):504–9.
45. Sung JY, Kuwabara S, Ogawara K, et al. Patterns of nerve conduction abnormal-ities in POEMS syndrome. Muscle Nerve 2002;26(2):189–93.
46. Min JH, Hong YH, Lee KW. Electrophysiological features of patients with POEMS syndrome. Clin Neurophysiol 2005;116(4):965–8.
47. Mauermann ML, Sorenson EJ, Dispenzieri A, et al. Uniform demyelination and more severe axonal loss distinguish POEMS syndrome from CIDP. J Neurol Neu-rosurg Psychiatry 2012;83(5):480–6.
48. Vital C, Vital A, Ferrer X, et al. Crow-Fukase (POEMS) syndrome: a study of pe-ripheral nerve biopsy in five new cases. J Peripher Nerv Syst 2003;8(3):136–44.
49. Orefice G, Morra VB, De Michele G, et al. POEMS syndrome: clinical, patholog-ical and immunological study of a case. Neurol Res 1994;16(6):477–80.
50. Crisci C, Barbieri F, Parente D, et al. POEMS syndrome: follow-up study of a case. Clin Neurol Neurosurg 1992;94(1):65–8.

51. Bergouignan FX, Massonnat R, Vital C, et al. Uncompacted lamellae in three patients with POEMS syndrome. Eur Neurol 1987;27(3):173–81.
52. Khuda SE, Loo WM, Janz S, et al. Deregulation of c-Myc confers distinct survival requirements for memory B cells, plasma cells, and their progenitors. J Immunol 2008;181(11):7537–49.
53. Soubrier M, Labauge P, Jouanel P, et al. Restricted use of Vlambda genes in POEMS syndrome. Haematologica 2004;89(4):ECR02.
54. Nakaseko C, Abe D, Takeuchi M, et al. Restricted oligo-clonal usage of monoclonal immunoglobulin {lambda} light chain germline in POEMS syndrome. ASH Annual Meeting Abstracts 2007;110(11):2483.
55. Aravamudan B, Tong C, Lacy MQ, et al. Immunoglobulin variable light chain restriction, cytokine expression and plasma cell-stromal cell interactions in POEMS syndrome patients. ASH Annual Meeting Abstracts 2008;112(11):2744.
56. Kang WY, Shen KN, Duan MH, et al. 14q32 translocations and 13q14 deletions are common cytogenetic abnormalities in POEMS syndrome. Eur J Haematol 2013;91(6):490–6.
57. Bryce AH, Ketterling RP, Gertz MA, et al. A novel report of cig-FISH and cytogenetics in POEMS syndrome. Am J Hematol 2008;83(11):840–1.
58. Tanaka O, Ohsawa T. The POEMS syndrome: report of three cases with radiographic abnormalities. Radiologe 1984;24(10):472–4.
59. Chong ST, Beasley HS, Daffner RH. POEMS syndrome: radiographic appearance with MRI correlation. Skeletal Radiol 2006;35(9):690–5.
60. Pan Q, Li J, Li F, et al. Characterizing POEMS syndrome with 18F-fludeoxyglucose positron emission tomography/computed tomography. J Nucl Med 2015; 56(9):1334–7.
61. Cui RT, Yu SY, Huang XS, et al. The characteristics of ascites in patients with POEMS syndrome. Ann Hematol 2013;92(12):1661–4.
62. Tokashiki T, Hashiguchi T, Arimura K, et al. Predictive value of serial platelet count and VEGF determination for the management of DIC in the Crow-Fukase (POEMS) syndrome. Intern Med 2003;42(12):1240–3.
63. Endo I, Mitsui T, Nishino M, et al. Diurnal fluctuation of edema synchronized with plasma VEGF concentration in a patient with POEMS syndrome. Intern Med 2002;41(12):1196–8.
64. Nakano A, Mitsui T, Endo I, et al. Solitary plasmacytoma with VEGF overproduction: report of a patient with polyneuropathy. Neurology 2001;56(6):818–9.
65. Wang C, Zhou YL, Cai H, et al. Markedly elevated serum total N-terminal propeptide of type I collagen is a novel marker for the diagnosis and follow up of patients with POEMS syndrome. Haematologica 2014;99(6):e78–80.
66. Ghandi GY, Basu R, Dispenzieri A, et al. Endocrinopathy in POEMS syndrome: the Mayo Clinic experience. Mayo Clin Proc 2007;82(7):836–42.
67. Dispenzieri A, Moreno-Aspitia A, Lacy MQ, et al. Peripheral blood stem cell transplant (PBSCT) in a large series of patients with POEMS syndrome. Biol Blood Marrow Transplant 2004;10(2):14–5.
68. Shirabe S, Kishikawa M, Mine M, et al. Crow-Fukase syndrome associated with extramedullary plasmacytoma [review] [11 refs]. Jpn J Med 1991;30(1):64–6.
69. Thajeb P, Chee CY, Lo SF, et al. The POEMS syndrome among Chinese: association with Castleman's disease and some immunological abnormalities. Acta Neurol Scand 1989;80(6):492–500.
70. Papo T, Soubrier M, Marcelin AG, et al. Human herpesvirus 8 infection, Castleman's disease and POEMS syndrome [letter]. Br J Haematol 1999;104(4):932–3.

71. Vital C, Gherardi R, Vital A, et al. Uncompacted myelin lamellae in polyneuropathy, organomegaly, endocrinopathy, M-protein and skin changes syndrome. Ultrastructural study of peripheral nerve biopsy from 22 patients. Acta Neuropathol 1994;87(3):302–7.

72. Yang SG, Cho KH, Bang YJ, et al. A case of glomeruloid hemangioma associated with multicentric Castleman's disease. Am J Dermatopathol 1998;20(3):266–70.

73. Kobayashi H, Ii K, Sano T, et al. Plasma-cell dyscrasia with polyneuropathy and endocrine disorders associated with dysfunction of salivary glands. Am J Surg Pathol 1985;9(10):759–63.

74. Bitter M, Komaiko W, Franklin W. Giant lymph node hyperplasia with osteoblastic bone lesions and the POEMS (Takatsuki's) syndrome. Cancer 1985;56:188–94.

75. Lapresle J, Lacroix-Ciaudo C, Reynes M, et al. Crow-Fukase syndrome (POEMS syndrome) and osseous mastocytosis secondary to Castleman's angiofollicular lymphoid hyperplasia. Rev Neurol (Paris) 1986;142(10):731–7 [in French].

76. Gherardi R, Baudrimont M, Kujas M, et al. Pathological findings in three non-Japanese patients with the POEMS syndrome. Virchows Arch A Pathol Anat Histopathol 1988;413(4):357–65.

77. Dworak O, Tschubel K, Zhou H, et al. Angiofollicular lymphatic hyperplasia with plasmacytoma and polyneuropathy: a case report with immunohistochemical study. Klin Wochenschr 1988;66(13):591–5 [in German].

78. Rolon PG, Audouin J, Diebold J, et al. Multicentric angiofollicular lymph node hyperplasia associated with a solitary osteolytic costal IgG lambda myeloma. POEMS syndrome in a South American (Paraguayan) patient. Pathol Res Pract 1989;185(4):468–75.

79. Carcaterra A, Santini R, Sozzi G, et al. Crow-Fukase syndrome (POEMS syndrome). The first Italian presentation of a case and review of the literature [review] [33 refs]. G Ital Dermatol Venereol 1990;125(3):97–103 [in Italian].

80. Chan JK, Fletcher CD, Hicklin GA, et al. Glomeruloid hemangioma. A distinctive cutaneous lesion of multicentric Castleman's disease associated with POEMS syndrome. Am J Surg Pathol 1990;14(11):1036–46.

81. Brazis PW, Liesegang TJ, Bolling JP, et al. When do optic disc edema and peripheral neuropathy constitute poetry? Surv Ophthalmol 1990;35(3):219–25.

82. Munoz G, Geijo P, Moldenhauer F, et al. Plasmacellular Castleman's disease and POEMS syndrome. Histopathology 1990;17(2):172–4.

83. Gherardi RK, Malapert D, Degos JD. Castleman disease-POEMS syndrome overlap [letter; comment]. Ann Intern Med 1991;114(6):520–1.

84. Myers BM, Miralles GD, Taylor CA, et al. POEMS syndrome with idiopathic flushing mimicking carcinoid syndrome. Am J Med 1991;90(5):646–8.

85. Coto V, Auletta M, Oliviero U, et al. POEMS syndrome: an Italian case with diagnostic and therapeutic implications. Ann Ital Med Int 1991;6(4):416–9.

86. Bosco J, Pathmanathan R. POEMS syndrome, osteosclerotic myeloma and Castleman's disease: a case report. Aust N Z J Med 1991;21(4):454–6.

87. Mandler RN, Kerrigan DP, Smart J, et al. Castleman's disease in POEMS syndrome with elevated interleukin-6 [see comments]. Cancer 1992;69(11):2697–703.

88. Nakazawa K, Itoh N, Shigematsu H, et al. An autopsy case of Crow-Fukase (POEMS) syndrome with a high level of IL-6 in the ascites. Special reference to glomerular lesions. Acta Pathol Jpn 1992;42(9):651–6.

89. Emile C, Danon F, Fermand JP, et al. Castleman disease in POEMS syndrome with elevated interleukin-6 [letter; comment]. Cancer 1993;71(3):874.

90. Judge MR, McGibbon DH, Thompson RP. Angioendotheliomatosis associated with Castleman's lymphoma and POEMS syndrome. Clin Exp Dermatol 1993; 18(4):360–2.
91. Del Rio R, Alsina M, Monteagudo J, et al. POEMS syndrome and multiple angioproliferative lesions mimicking generalized histiocytomas. Acta Derm Venereol 1994;74(5):388–90.
92. Bhatia M, Maheshwari MC. Angiofollicular lymphoid hyperplasia presenting as POEMS syndrome. J Assoc Physicians India 1994;42(9):751–2.
93. Adelman HM, Cacciatore ML, Pascual JF, et al. Case report: Castleman disease in association with POEMS. Am J Med Sci 1994;307(2):112–4.
94. Pareyson D, Marazzi R, Confalonieri P, et al. The POEMS syndrome: report of six cases. Ital J Neurol Sci 1994;15(7):353–8.
95. Ku A, Lachmann E, Tunkel R, et al. Severe polyneuropathy: initial manifestation of Castleman's disease associated with POEMS syndrome. Arch Phys Med Rehabil 1995;76(7):692–4.
96. Huang CC, Chu CC. Poor response to intravenous immunoglobulin therapy in patients with Castleman's disease and the POEMS syndrome [letter; comment]. J Neurol 1996;243(10):726–7.
97. Chang YJ, Huang CC, Chu CC. Intravenous immunoglobulin therapy in POEMS syndrome: a case report. Zhonghua Yi Xue Za Zhi (Taipei) 1996;58(5):366–9.
98. Forster A, Muri R. Recurrent cerebrovascular insult–manifestation of POEMS syndrome? Schweiz Med Wochenschr 1998;128(26):1059–64 [in German].
99. Belec L, Mohamed AS, Authier FJ, et al. Human herpesvirus 8 infection in patients with POEMS syndrome-associated multicentric Castleman's disease. Blood 1999;93(11):3643–53.
100. Belec L, Authier FJ, Mohamed AS, et al. Antibodies to human herpesvirus 8 in POEMS (polyneuropathy, organomegaly, endocrinopathy, M protein, skin changes) syndrome with multicentric Castleman's disease. Clin Infect Dis 1999;28(3):678–9.
101. Singh D, Wadhwa J, Kumar L, et al. POEMS syndrome: experience with fourteen cases. Leuk Lymphoma 2003;44(10):1749–52.
102. Zhang B, Song X, Liang B, et al. The clinical study of POEMS syndrome in China. Neuro Endocrinol Lett 2010;31(2):229–37.
103. Kulkarni GB, Mahadevan A, Taly AB, et al. Clinicopathological profile of polyneuropathy, organomegaly, endocrinopathy, M protein and skin changes (POEMS) syndrome. J Clin Neurosci 2011;18(3):356–60.
104. Barete S, Mouawad R, Choquet S, et al. Skin manifestations and vascular endothelial growth factor levels in POEMS syndrome: impact of autologous hematopoietic stem cell transplantation. Arch Dermatol 2010;146(6):615–23.
105. Bachmeyer C. Acquired facial atrophy: a neglected clinical sign of POEMS syndrome. Am J Hematol 2012;87(1):131.
106. Lee FY, Chiu HC. POEMS syndrome with calciphylaxis: a case report. Acta Derm Venereol 2011;91(1):96–7.
107. De Roma I, Filotico R, Cea M, et al. Calciphylaxis in a patient with POEMS syndrome without renal failure and/or hyperparathyroidism. A case report. Ann Ital Med Int 2004;19(4):283–7.
108. Allam JS, Kennedy CC, Aksamit TR, et al. Pulmonary manifestations in patients with POEMS syndrome: a retrospective review of 137 patients. Chest 2008; 133(4):969–74.
109. Ishikawa O, Nihei Y, Ishikawa H. The skin changes of POEMS syndrome. Br J Dermatol 1987;117(4):523–6.

110. Jitsukawa K, Hayashi Y, Sato S, et al. Cutaneous angioma in Crow-Fukase syndrome: the nature of globules within the endothelial cells. J Dermatol 1988;15(6): 513–22.

111. Rongioletti F, Gambini C, Lerza R. Glomeruloid hemangioma. A cutaneous marker of POEMS syndrome. Am J Dermatopathol 1994;16(2):175–8.

112. Santoro L, Manganelli F, Bruno R, et al. Sural nerve and epidermal vascular abnormalities in a case of POEMS syndrome. Eur J Neurol 2006;13(1):99–102.

113. Kaushik M, Pulido JS, Abreu R, et al. Ocular findings in patients with polyneuropathy, organomegaly, endocrinopathy, monoclonal gammopathy, and skin changes syndrome. Ophthalmology 2011;118(4):778–82.

114. Cui R, Yu S, Huang X, et al. Papilloedema is an independent prognostic factor for POEMS syndrome. J Neurol 2014;261(1):60–5.

115. Lesprit P, Godeau B, Authier FJ, et al. Pulmonary hypertension in POEMS syndrome: a new feature mediated by cytokines. Am J Respir Crit Care Med 1998; 157(3 Pt 1):907–11.

116. Li J, Tian Z, Zheng HY, et al. Pulmonary hypertension in POEMS syndrome. Haematologica 2013;98(3):393–8.

117. Stankowski-Drengler T, Gertz MA, Katzmann JA, et al. Serum immunoglobulin free light chain measurements and heavy chain isotype usage provide insight into disease biology in patients with POEMS syndrome. Am J Hematol 2010; 85(6):431–4.

118. Ye W, Wang C, Cai QQ, et al. Renal impairment in patients with polyneuropathy, organomegaly, endocrinopathy, monoclonal gammopathy and skin changes syndrome: incidence, treatment and outcome. Nephrol Dial Transplant 2016; 31(2):275–83.

119. Sanada S, Ookawara S, Karube H, et al. Marked recovery of severe renal lesions in POEMS syndrome with high-dose melphalan therapy supported by autologous blood stem cell transplantation. Am J Kidney Dis 2006;47(4):672–9.

120. Navis GJ, Dullaart RP, Vellenga E, et al. Renal disease in POEMS syndrome: report on a case and review of the literature [review] [25 refs]. Nephrol Dial Transplant 1994;9(10):1477–81.

121. Viard JP, Lesavre P, Boitard C, et al. POEMS syndrome presenting as systemic sclerosis. Clinical and pathologic study of a case with microangiopathic glomerular lesions. Am J Med 1988;84(3 Pt 1):524–8.

122. Sano M, Terasaki T, Koyama A, et al. Glomerular lesions associated with the Crow-Fukase syndrome. Virchows Arch A Pathol Anat Histopathol 1986; 409(1):3–9.

123. Takazoe K, Shimada T, Kawamura T, et al. Possible mechanism of progressive renal failure in Crow-Fukase syndrome [letter]. Clin Nephrol 1997;47(1):66–7.

124. Mizuiri S, Mitsuo K, Sakai K, et al. Renal involvement in POEMS syndrome. Nephron 1991;59(1):153–6.

125. Stewart PM, McIntyre MA, Edwards CR. The endocrinopathy of POEMS syndrome. Scott Med J 1989;34(5):520–2.

126. Nakamoto Y, Imai H, Yasuda T, et al. A spectrum of clinicopathological features of nephropathy associated with POEMS syndrome. Nephrol Dial Transplant 1999;14(10):2370–8.

127. Fukatsu A, Ito Y, Yuzawa Y, et al. A case of POEMS syndrome showing elevated serum interleukin 6 and abnormal expression of interleukin 6 in the kidney. Nephron 1992;62(1):47–51.

128. Lesprit P, Authier FJ, Gherardi R, et al. Acute arterial obliteration: a new feature of the POEMS syndrome? Medicine (Baltimore) 1996;75(4):226–32.

129. Dispenzieri A. POEMS syndrome. Blood Rev 2007;21(6):285–99.
130. Zenone T, Bastion Y, Salles G, et al. POEMS syndrome, arterial thrombosis and thrombocythaemia. J Intern Med 1996;240(2):107–9.
131. Soubrier M, Guillon R, Dubost JJ, et al. Arterial obliteration in POEMS syndrome: possible role of vascular endothelial growth factor. J Rheumatol 1998;25(4): 813–5.
132. Bova G, Pasqui AL, Saletti M, et al. POEMS syndrome with vascular lesions: a role for interleukin-1beta and interleukin-6 increase–a case report. Angiology 1998;49(11):937–40.
133. Kang K, Chu K, Kim DE, et al. POEMS syndrome associated with ischemic stroke. Arch Neurol 2003;60(5):745–9.
134. Dupont SA, Dispenzieri A, Mauermann ML, et al. Cerebral infarction in POEMS syndrome: incidence, risk factors, and imaging characteristics. Neurology 2009; 73(16):1308–12.
135. Atsumi T, Kato K, Kurosawa S, et al. A case of Crow-Fukase syndrome with elevated soluble interleukin-6 receptor in cerebrospinal fluid. Response to double-filtration plasmapheresis and corticosteroids. Acta Haematol 1995; 94(2):90–4.
136. Gaba AR, Stein RS, Sweet DL, et al. Multicentric giant lymph node hyperplasia. Am J Clin Pathol 1978;69(1):86–90.
137. Hineman VL, Phyliky RL, Banks PM. Angiofollicular lymph node hyperplasia and peripheral neuropathy: association with monoclonal gammopathy. Mayo Clin Proc 1982;57(6):379–82.
138. Black DA, Forgacs I, Davies DR, et al. Pseudotumour cerebri in a patient with Castleman's disease. Postgrad Med J 1988;64(749):217–9.
139. Feigert JM, Sweet DL, Coleman M, et al. Multicentric angiofollicular lymph node hyperplasia with peripheral neuropathy, pseudotumor cerebri, IgA dysproteine- mia, and thrombocytosis in women. A distinct syndrome [see comments]. Ann Intern Med 1990;113(5):362–7.
140. Menke DM, Tiemann M, Camoriano JK, et al. Diagnosis of Castleman's disease by identification of an immunophenotypically aberrant population of mantle zone B lymphocytes in paraffin-embedded lymph node biopsies. Am J Clin Pathol 1996;105(3):268–76.
141. Mallory A, Spink WW. Angiomatous lymphoid hamartoma in the retroperitoneum presenting with neurologic signs in the legs. Ann Intern Med 1968;69(2):305–8.
142. Anonymous. Case records of the Massachusetts General Hospital. Weekly clin- icopathological exercises. Case 10-1987. A 59-year-old woman with progres- sive polyneuropathy and monoclonal gammopathy. N Engl J Med 1987; 316(10):606–18.
143. Yu GS, Carson JW. Giant lymph-node hyperplasia, plasma-cell type, of the mediastinum, with peripheral neuropathy. Am J Clin Pathol 1976;66(1):46–53.
144. Weisenburger DD, Nathwani BN, Winberg CD, et al. Multicentric angiofollicular lymph node hyperplasia: a clinicopathologic study of 16 cases. Hum Pathol 1985;16(2):162–72.
145. Donaghy M, Hall P, Gawler J, et al. Peripheral neuropathy associated with Cas- tleman's disease. J Neurol Sci 1989;89:253–67.
146. Ganti AK, Pipinos I, Culcea E, et al. Successful hematopoietic stem-cell trans- plantation in multicentric Castleman disease complicated by POEMS syndrome. Am J Hematol 2005;79(3):206–10.

147. Menke DM, Camoriano JK, Banks PM. Angiofollicular lymph node hyperplasia: a comparison of unicentric, multicentric, hyaline vascular, and plasma cell types of disease by morphometric and clinical analysis. Mod Pathol 1992;5(5):525–30.

148. Naddaf E, Dispenzieri A, Mandrekar J, et al. Thrombocytosis distinguishes poems syndrome from chronic inflammatory demyelinating polyneuropathy. Muscle Nerve 2015;52(4):658–9.

149. Wong VA, Wade NK. POEMS syndrome: an unusual cause of bilateral optic disk swelling. Am J Ophthalmol 1998;126(3):452–4.

150. Hogan WJ, Lacy MQ, Wiseman GA, et al. Successful treatment of POEMS syndrome with autologous hematopoietic progenitor cell transplantation. Bone Marrow Transplant 2001;28(3):305–9.

151. Rovira M, Carreras E, Blade J, et al. Dramatic improvement of POEMS syndrome following autologous haematopoietic cell transplantation. Br J Haematol 2001; 115(2):373–5.

152. Jaccard A, Royer B, Bordessoule D, et al. High-dose therapy and autologous blood stem cell transplantation in POEMS syndrome. Blood 2002;99(8):3057–9.

153. Peggs KS, Paneesha S, Kottaridis PD, et al. Peripheral blood stem cell transplantation for POEMS syndrome. Bone Marrow Transplant 2002;30(6):401–4.

154. Soubrier M, Ruivard M, Dubost JJ, et al. Successful use of autologous bone marrow transplantation in treating a patient with POEMS syndrome. Bone Marrow Transplant 2002;30(1):61–2.

155. Wiesmann A, Weissert R, Kanz L, et al. Long-term follow-up on a patient with incomplete POEMS syndrome undergoing high-dose therapy and autologous blood stem cell transplantation. Blood 2002;100(7):2679–80.

156. Dispenzieri A, Kyle RA, Lacy MQ, et al. Superior survival in primary systemic amyloidosis patients undergoing peripheral blood stem cell transplantation: a case-control study. Blood 2004;103(10):3960–3.

157. Takai K, Niikuni K, Kurasaki T. Successful treatment of POEMS syndrome with high-dose chemotherapy and autologous peripheral blood stem cell transplantation. Rinsho Ketsueki 2004;45(10):1111–4 [in Japanese].

158. Kastritis E, Terpos E, Anagnostopoulos A, et al. Angiogenetic factors and biochemical markers of bone metabolism in POEMS syndrome treated with high-dose therapy and autologous stem cell support. Clin Lymphoma Myeloma 2006;7(1):73–6.

159. Kuwabara S, Misawa S, Kanai K, et al. Autologous peripheral blood stem cell transplantation for POEMS syndrome. Neurology 2006;66(1):105–7.

160. Kojima H, Katsuoka Y, Katsura Y, et al. Successful treatment of a patient with POEMS syndrome by tandem high-dose chemotherapy with autologous CD34+ purged stem cell rescue. Int J Hematol 2006;84(2):182–5.

161. Imai N, Kitamura E, Tachibana T, et al. Efficacy of autologous peripheral blood stem cell transplantation in POEMS syndrome with polyneuropathy. Intern Med 2007;46(3):135–8.

162. Davis L, Drachman D. Myeloma neuropathy. Successful treatment of two patients and review of cases. Arch Neurol 1972;27(6):507–11.

163. Kuwabara S, Hattori T, Shimoe Y, et al. Long term melphalan-prednisolone chemotherapy for POEMS syndrome. J Neurol Neurosurg Psychiatry 1997; 63(3):385–7.

164. Arima F, Dohmen K, Yamano Y, et al. Five cases of Crow-Fukase syndrome. Fukuoka Igaku Zasshi 1992;83(2):112–20 [in Japanese].

165. Barrier JH, Le Noan H, Mussini JM, et al. Stabilisation of a severe case of P.O.E.M.S. syndrome after tamoxifen administration [letter]. J Neurol Neurosurg Psychiatry 1989;52(2):286.
166. Matsui H, Udaka F, Kubori T, et al. POEMS syndrome demonstrating VEGF decrease by ticlopidine. Intern Med 2004;43(11):1082–3.
167. Authier FJ, Belec L, Levy Y, et al. All-trans-retinoic acid in POEMS syndrome. Therapeutic effect associated with decreased circulating levels of proinflammatory cytokines. Arthritis Rheum 1996;39(8):1423–6.
168. Sternberg AJ, Davies P, Macmillan C, et al. Strontium-89: a novel treatment for a case of osteosclerotic myeloma associated with life-threatening neuropathy. Br J Haematol 2002;118(3):821–4.
169. Kim SY, Lee SA, Ryoo HM, et al. Thalidomide for POEMS syndrome. Ann Hematol 2006;85(8):545–6.
170. Sinisalo M, Hietaharju A, Sauranen J, et al. Thalidomide in POEMS syndrome: case report. Am J Hematol 2004;76(1):66–8.
171. Badros A, Porter N, Zimrin A. Bevacizumab therapy for POEMS syndrome. Blood 2005;106(3):1135.
172. Straume O, Bergheim J, Ernst P. Bevacizumab therapy for POEMS syndrome. Blood 2006;107(12):4972–3 [author reply: 4973–4].
173. Dispenzieri A, Klein CJ, Mauermann ML. Lenalidomide therapy in a patient with POEMS syndrome. Blood 2007;110(3):1075–6.

POEMS Syndrome
Therapeutic Options

Arnaud Jaccard, MD, PhD

KEYWORDS

- POEMS syndrome • Autologous stem cell transplantation • VEGF • Lenalidomide
- Thalidomide • Bortezomib

KEY POINTS

- The aim of polyneuropathy, organomegaly, endocrinopathy, monoclonal gammopathy, and skin changes (POEMS) syndrome treatment is to target the underlying plasma cell clone with a risk-adapted therapy based on the extent of the plasma cell disorder.
- Eradication by radiation or surgery of a localized lesion can improve the symptoms of POEMS syndrome and also be curative.
- High-dose chemotherapy with autologous stem cell transplantation is the treatment of choice for fit patients with a disseminated disease.
- Lenalidomide, thalidomide, and bortezomib are promising treatments.
- Lenalidomide and dexamethasone may be used before high-dose therapy and radiation to get rapid neurologic improvement and to prevent engraftment syndrome.

INTRODUCTION

Treatment of the polyneuropathy, organomegaly, endocrinopathy, monoclonal gammopathy, and skin changes (POEMS) syndrome can be broken down into 3 major categories: targeting the underlying clone; targeting the cytokines, particularly vascular endothelial growth factor (VEGF), that may be responsible for many clinical manifestations of the syndrome; and supportive care, mostly aimed at improving patients' neurologic status.

There are very few prospective studies on the treatment of this rare disease; recommendations on treatment have to be made essentially from retrospective studies and case reports, even if recently some prospective studies have been published,[1,2] one of them being a randomized one,[2] but with very few patients.

Targeting the underlying clone, which is most of the time a plasma cell clone, is the most important part of the treatment. Indeed, eradication by radiation or surgery of a

Disclosure Statement: Janssen and Celgene, honoraria and research support.
Department of Clinical Hematology, Reference Center for AL Amyloidosis, CHU, 2 Avenue ML King, Limoges 87000, France
E-mail address: arnaud.jaccard@chu-limoges.fr

Hematol Oncol Clin N Am 32 (2018) 141–151
https://doi.org/10.1016/j.hoc.2017.09.011
hemonc.theclinics.com

localized lesion can improve the symptoms of POEMS syndrome but also be curative, highlighting the role of the B-cell dyscrasia in the pathogenesis of this disease. POEMS syndrome could be considered as a monoclonal gammopathy of clinical significance (MGCS)[3] whereby all the damages are not linked to the tumoral mass but to a toxic clone, often small,[4] which produces a monoclonal immunoglobulin, complete or heavy or light chain only, responsible for the symptoms. In POEMS syndrome, the toxic protein seems to be a monoclonal lambda light chain encoded by only 2 lambda light chain variable genes (IGVL1) able to drive the synthesis of huge amounts of VEGF by an unknown mechanism.[5–8] As in other MGCS, to give the most accurate treatment of the underlying clone is of paramount importance.

UNDERLYING HEMOPATHY

In most cases, there is a subtle plasma cell proliferation, rarely the cause of bone pains or hypercalcemia; the treatment will be adapted from myeloma if disseminated or bone plasmocytoma if localized. In two-thirds of cases there is an often-minimal and difficult-to-highlight bone marrow involvement (median percent of plasma cells <5%).[9] As a simple myelogram is not sensitive enough to detect this small infiltration, either a bone marrow biopsy with immunohistochemical staining or a bone marrow aspiration with flow cytometry have to be performed, with the biopsy being apparently more accurate because it can also show typical lymphoid aggregates with plasma cell rimming, which helps in making the diagnosis.[9]

A monoclonal immunoglobulin can be detected with immuno-fixation in about 80% of patients, immunoglobulin A (IgA) slightly more often than IgG, with only a small percentage of patients having a monoclonal IgM or an isolated monoclonal light chain. The levels of monoclonal immunoglobulin are generally not very high, with a median level of 10 g/L. The presence of 2 clones is not rare, and a polyclonal hypergammaglobulinemia leading to a nonspecific increase of serum monoclonal free light chains can often be found. With the dosage of free light chains, most patients experience an increase in the lambda light chain; but in 80% of cases, the kappa/lambda ratio stays normal.[10]

Some patients have the equivalent of a monoclonal immunoglobulin of undetermined signification; as in amyloid light-chain (AL) amyloidosis, the treatment should be different if this is an IgM or another isotype. A small number of them have a lymphoplasmocytic proliferation often associated with a monoclonal IgM.[11] Finally, some of them have a chronic lymphocytic leukemia or a lymphoma. Every time, the histologic aspect is unusual, probably because of the abnormal production of VEGF and other cytokines.

SPECIFIC TREATMENTS

A treatment algorithm has been proposed by Angela Dispenzieri[12,13] (**Fig. 1**). It relies on the existence or absence of bone marrow involvement searched by bone marrow biopsy and on the existence of one or several bone lesions. If there is no medullar infiltration, then a search for bone lesions susceptible to irradiation is essential using all available tools: bone radiography, MRI, computed tomography (CT) scanner, bone scintigraphy, and PET scan. It is not completely clear which tool is most accurate. Low-dose whole-body CT scan, like what is now widely used in multiple myeloma instead of classic bone radiographies, is useful to detect all bone lesions and also other features of the disease, pleura effusions, ascites, adenopathies, and hepatosplenomegaly. PET scan is also used, but fludeoxyglucose (FDG) uptake can be variable. It could be useful to assess the response to treatment and to guide radiation on residual lesions.

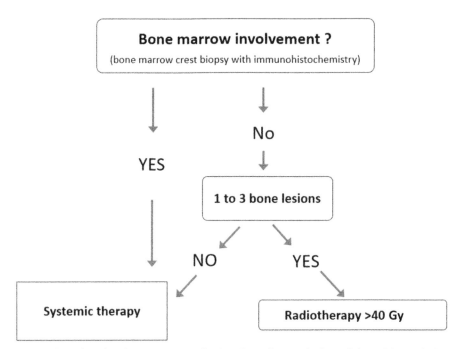

Fig. 1. Algorithm for the treatment of POEMS syndrome. (*Adapted from* Dispenzieri A. POEMS syndrome: 2017 update on diagnosis, risk stratification, and management. Am J Hematol 2017;92(8):821; with permission.)

TREATMENT WHEN THERE ARE 1 TO 3 BONE LESIONS AND NO DISSEMINATED BONE MARROW INVOLVEMENT

Patients with no medullar infiltration and with a limited number of bone lesions that can be treated by radiation should receive curative radiation, doses of 40 Gy or more, as it is indicated for solitary bone plasmacytoma.[14] After radiation, the symptoms of POEMS syndrome slowly improve, typically after an initial worsening, in more than half of the patients, with some patients probably being cured. A series of 38 Mayo Clinic patients who received radiotherapy as first-line treatment was published in 2012 with a median follow-up of 43 months and showed a 4-year survival rate of 97% and a 4-year failure-free survival rate of 52%, with most relapses or nonresponses happening within the first year.[15] Nearly 40% of the cohort had more than 1 bone lesion without any clear difference in risk of relapse or progression in patients with 1 or 3 lesions. An update of this series with 83 patients was published in 2016,[16] the 6-year progression-free survival was 62%. In a small series from South Korea,[17] 13 patients were treated by radiotherapy as the first-line treatment (n = 6) or as a consolidative treatment (n = 7). The results were comparable with that of the Mayo series; interestingly, radiotherapy was effective in improving POEMS syndrome–associated symptoms in some patients who did not respond to chemotherapy.

Because neuropathy typically takes approximately 3 months to stabilize and 6 months to begin to improve after radiotherapy,[15] unnecessary additional treatment is sometimes given to the patients. Evaluation after radiotherapy should take into account not only clinical symptoms but also VEGF levels, hematologic response, and FDG-PET/CT scan (**Fig. 2**).

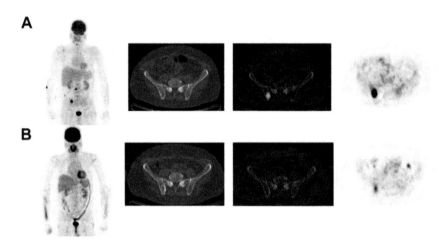

Fig. 2. FDG-PET/CT scan before and after treatment. A 59-year-old patient relapsing 5 years after autologous stem cell transplant. FDG-PET/CT scan (*A*) at relapse and (*B*) after 5 cycles of lenalidomide and dexamethasone showing a partial response.

Patients with advanced disease, particularly with a severe neuropathy or rapidly deteriorating, should receive an adjuvant therapy waiting for radiotherapy efficacy. Corticosteroids, for example, dexamethasone 40 mg for 4 days every 2 weeks, usually improve POEMS-related symptoms. A short course of lenalidomide and dexamethasone before radiotherapy may provide a very rapid neurologic improvement,[18] and this strategy is tested in a French prospective trial (**Fig. 3**).

TREATMENT WHEN THERE IS DISSEMINATED BONE MARROW INVOLVEMENT OR NO BONE LESION OR MANY BONE LESIONS

Patients with medullar involvement or patients without medullar involvement but also without specific bone lesions or more than 3 bone lesions should receive a systemic treatment targeting the underlying clone. In few cases with a very small percentage of plasma cells in the bone marrow and with a large plasmacytoma, radiation can be

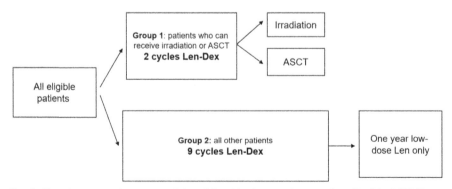

Fig. 3. French prospective protocol: lenalidomide-dexamethasone (Len-Dex) in POEMS syndrome. Len: 25 mg 21 days/28 (10 mg if creatinine clearance <50 mL/mn). Dex: 40 mg/wk (20 mg if aged >75 years or frail). Low-dose Len: 10 mg 28 days/28 for 12 cycles. Aspirin or low molecular weight heparin. ASCT, autologous stem cell transplant.

considered but is not expected to be curative. More often radiation will be proposed as an adjuvant therapy after some months, in case of an insufficient response.

The first treatment to show quasi-consistent effectiveness is high-dose chemotherapy with autologous stem cell transplant (ASCT). The first series of patients was published in 2002[19]; several others have later confirmed that ASCT is quite effective in this disease,[20–22] with nearly 100% of patients having a hematologic and neurologic response and excellent survival. Mortality linked to intensive treatment is not high, but intensive treatment seems to come along with a worrying number of complications in POEMS syndrome compared with myeloma, particularly engraftment syndrome,[23] combining fever, weight gain, cutaneous eruptions, diarrhea, and respiratory signs occurring between 7 and 15 days after stem cell infusion. A short course of corticosteroid should be rapidly given if these signs appear, usually with a rapid resolution of symptoms.

Patients with POEMS syndrome have a low tumor burden and usually a nonproliferating plasma cell clone, and induction chemotherapy is not mandatory; but the author's experience is that 1 cycle of dexamethasone 40 mg daily for 4 days before the stem-cell collection and between collection and ASCT may prevent engraftment syndrome. It has also been shown that thalidomide and lenalidomide treatment before ASCT is able to prevent this syndrome.[18,24] Treatments with these drugs also have the advantage of giving a rapid response, (cf infra) allowing patients to undergo ASCT in better shape. In most cases, the conditioning has been high-dose melphalan, 140 to 200 mg/m^2. Some patients relapse; but after a 5-year follow-up, 75% of patients are still responding.[21,22] Some rare patients with a high percentage of plasma cells in the bone marrow have relapsed within 2 years. In their long follow-up of patients who were treated with ASCT, the Mayo Clinic team[21] found that IgG lambda monoclonal components compared with IgA and FDG-avid lesions on the baseline PET scan are risk factors for progression.

When neither of these two options is possible (no localized lesion or patients too old or too frail to receive intensive treatment), there is no consensus on the best strategy. Treatment is mainly derived from other plasma cell disorders, myeloma, and AL amyloidosis. **Table 1** is a summary of treatments used in POEMS syndrome with their outcome.

Table 1
Different treatments used in POEMS syndrome

Regimen	Conditions	Outcome
Radiotherapy	1–3 bone lesions, no bone marrow involvement	>50% response[15,17]
Melphalan-dexamethasone	Unfit for ASCT	100% VEGF and neurologic response[1]
ASCT	Fit patients, successful collection of stem cells	100% of surviving patients have a response[19–21]
Thalidomide-dexamethasone	No previous arterial event	VEGF response but risk of toxic neuropathy[2,3,24]
Lenalidomide-dexamethasone	No previous arterial event	VEGF and rapid neurologic response, seems effective before radiation or ASCT[18,25–28]
Bortezomib-containing regimens	Usually in second line	88% of VEGF response, 95% of neurologic improvement[30,32]

Corticosteroids are effective to a certain extent but remain inconsistent and generally insufficient. Some of the features of the syndrome, such as pulmonary hypertension, may be very sensitive to corticosteroids.[31]

Alkylating agents have been widely used in POEMS syndrome. A prospective trial using the association of melphalan and dexamethasone, inspired by the AL amyloidosis experience, has been published.[1] It included 31 patients who received 12 cycles; 81% of them had a hematologic response, and all of them experienced a decrease in VEGF accompanied by a neurologic improvement. These results, yielded by a short series with a relatively short follow-up, must be confirmed. Cyclophosphamide-based therapy, with dexamethasone or proteasome inhibitors, has been also used with good results.[13]

Numerous other treatments have been tested. The use of anti-VEGF antibodies was logical given the role of this cytokine in POEMS syndrome. The first reported cases seemingly showed the decent effectiveness of bevacizumab, particularly in association with alkylating agents; but soon the cases of 3 patients who died in the weeks following its administration were published. One publication then reported 6 cases directly and gathered 11 more from the literature.[29] Out of these 17 patients treated with bevacizumab, 6 died in the weeks following its administration, which is very unusual in POEMS syndrome, as it is generally associated with a long life expectancy.[13] One hypothesis that could explain those deaths is the apoptosis induced by VEGF privation in hypertrophied endothelial cells after a long exposure to high levels of VEGF. This massive apoptosis would then trigger the destruction of the neovascularization inducing a capillary leak syndrome. Bevacizumab is, thus, a dangerous treatment of this disease and must not be used.

Other treatments used in myeloma have been tried in POEMS syndrome. More than 30 patients treated with a bortezomib-containing regimen have been reported as case records[30] or very recently as a retrospective study on 20 patients treated with a reduced dose of bortezomib (1 mg/m^2 intravenously on days 1, 4, 8, and 11), cyclophosphamide, and dexamethasone.[32] No neurologic worsening was observed in this series, although bortezomib was given twice a week and intravenously. With a median follow-up time of 11 months, the overall hematologic response rate was 76% with 7 patients achieving a complete hematologic response; 88% had a decrease in the VEGF serum level of more than 50%. Ninety-five percent of patients had an improvement of peripheral neuropathy.

Thalidomide has been used in Japan with neurologic improvements, a decrease in VEGF, and a decrease in the frequency of engraftment syndrome when it was used before intensive treatments.[24] Of note it has been shown, associated with dexamethasone, in the only randomized trial done in this disease to date, more efficient than dexamethasone alone to reduce the VEGF level.[2] This interesting study only randomized 25 patients; the clinical results are not impressive enough to overcome the reluctance to propose this drug, with its well-known neurologic toxicity, as a first-line treatment.

Lenalidomide looks a lot more interesting because of its lack of neurologic toxicity, its effectiveness against plasma cells proliferations, and its anti-VEGF effect. The first case ever of a patient treated for a POEMS with lenalidomide was published in *Blood* in 2007.[26] It was the case of a 40-year-old man with disseminated POEMS syndrome, which had been evolving for 4 years, whose general condition was unfit for intensive treatment. He received 9 cycles of the association of lenalidomide (15 mg then 25 mg, 21 days a month) and weekly dexamethasone. This treatment was effective against the various clinical manifestations of POEMS, particularly neuropathy and edema, and led to a return of the serum VEGF levels to normal.

The author and colleagues have reported a retrospective series of 20 patients treated with lenalidomide and dexamethasone, 4 of whom were treatment naive and 16 of whom were nonresponding or relapsing.[27] All patients but one had a response, with a decrease in VEGF in the 17 patients who had an evaluation. A meta-analysis of lenalidomide collecting 19 publications, including the author and colleagues', and 51 patients have been published confirming these preliminary results.[28] A prospective study is currently in progress in France in which the patients receive 2 cycles of lenalidomide and dexamethasone, then an irradiation or intensive treatment if it is advisable or 9 cycles of lenalidomide and dexamethasone followed by 1 year of lenalidomide alone in small doses otherwise (see **Fig. 3**). Fifty patients have been included, and the first 27 patients have been reported at the American Society of Hematology's meeting in 2014.[18] The results confirm those obtained in the retrospective series with a hematologic and clinical response after 2 cycles in most patients and interestingly a very rapid neurologic response, unusual in this disease, possibly linked to the anti-VEGF effect of lenalidomide (**Table 2**). This association apparently also prevents the engraftment syndrome observed in intensive treatments, as was reported by Japanese investigators with thalidomide. Out of the 50 patients, 2 had a cerebrovascular accident, one of which was lethal. Arterial events are well known in POEMS syndrome; an article published in 2009 found a 13.5% risk of arterial events in a 5-year period in this disease, independently of treatment.[33] immunomodulatory drugs (IMiDs) should not be used in patients with a history of an arterial event and used with caution in patients with other risk factors, such as polycythemia or thrombocythemia. A prophylactic treatment of thromboses by aspirin and/or heparin of low molecular weight is essential.

No publication exists with the other treatments recently introduced in the therapeutic armamentarium in myeloma. The author and colleagues have used pomalidomide in some patients with encouraging results; it is probable that other new molecules, such as carfilzomib, ixazomib, or daratumumab, will have activity.

For patients with non–plasma-cell clones, treatment should be adapted to target the underlying disease, as it has been published for macroglobulinemia-associated POEMS syndrome.[11,34]

Many patients who initially have a diagnosis of chronic inflammatory demyelinating polyneuropathy have received intravenous immunoglobulin (IVIG) before the diagnosis of POEMS syndrome. IVIG or plasmapheresis is not really helpful in this disease[13] but may result in the reduction of serum VEGF[35] leading to a delay in diagnosis.

SECOND-LINE TREATMENT

In their study focusing on relapse and progression (R/P) after the initial treatment, Kourelis and colleagues[16] reported on 79 patients with a documented R/P among 291 patients with POEMS syndrome seen at the Mayo Clinic between 1974 and

Table 2	
French protocol with lenalidomide and dexamethasone, neurologic evaluation, 10-m walk test	
70-Year-Old Patient Who Walked with 2 Crutches at Inclusion	**65-Year-Old Patient with a Single Bone Lesion**
At inclusion: 17.0 s	At inclusion: 15.0 s
After 1 cycle: 12.6 s	After 1 cycle: 12.0 s
After 2 cycles: 9.90 s	After 2 cycles: 10.0 s
After 5 cycles: 8.20 s	After radiotherapy: 8.0 s

2014. Of note, one-third of the patients with an asymptomatic R/P were observed for a median of 9 months before initiating treatment. The investigators did not recommend initiating treatment in asymptomatic patients based only on VEGF elevation or with an isolated hematologic relapse. The author and colleagues' experience is that, in these patients, elevation of serum VEGF is often followed by a resurgence of symptoms, particularly neurologic manifestations, in the following weeks. So patients with an asymptomatic R/P should be monitored closely. For patients with symptomatic relapse or a positive PET scan, treatment should be given.

Patients with 1 to 2 dominant lesions on PET imaging and no progression in the bone marrow are eligible for radiation therapy. If a more extensive disease is present, then systemic therapy should be considered, depending on the initial treatment. As in myeloma, if R/P occurs a long time after initial treatment, it should be resumed; a second ASCT is feasible in young fit patients is possible. Long-term alkylating agents should be avoided taking into account the risk of myelodysplasia. Lenalidomide and dexamethasone or a bortezomib-containing regimen are possible options.

MONITORING RESPONSE

There is no consensus on what constitutes the criteria of the response to treatment in POEMS syndrome. Evaluating the hematologic response can prove difficult given the small size of the monoclonal peak often associated with a hypergammaglobulinemia and a normal ratio of light chains. In some patients, a very significant clinical benefit can be seen in the absence of an M-protein response. Monitoring the VEGF levels seems to be a much better way to predict the clinical response. It is not clear if serum or plasma measurement is more accurate. Measuring serum VEGF levels seems to be more sensitive for diagnosis, whereas it seems to be more accurate to assess the response in the plasma, with levels being much lower in plasma because of the release of VEGF contained within the platelets on clotting.[18,36]

Organ responses are difficult to assess when a multitude of organ systems are affected, and to date there are no defined criteria for organ responses. It has been proposed[37] to use a simplified organ response, which is limited to those systems causing the most morbidity, like peripheral neuropathy assessment, pulmonary function testing, and extravascular overload (grading ascites and pleural effusion as absent, mild, moderate, or severe). For neuropathy assessment, the most important criterion of clinical response in this disease, the Overall Neuropathy Limitations Scale, is a simple tool that is not perfect but can be easily used by the clinicians who are usually in charge of patients with POEMS syndrome.[38] Another simple test is the 10-minute walk test,[39] which can show a rapid response to treatment (see **Table 2**).

PROGNOSIS

In a report published in 2003,[40] when the median survival in myeloma was around 3 years, the median survival of a cohort of 99 patients was more than 13 years. With the introduction of new myeloma drugs and the frequent use of ASCT in this disease, the survival is clearly even better. A recent study from China including 362 patients found that a prognostic score can be made with 4 easily determined parameters to stratify patients: age greater than 50 years, presence of pulmonary hypertension, presence of pleural effusions, and estimated glomerular filtration rate less than 30 mL/min/1.73 m^2.[41] The 5-year overall survival in low- and high-risk groups was 100% and 71%, respectively, in the derivation cohort and 95% and 63% in the validation cohort. This score has been validated in a Mayo Clinic cohort of 138 patients[42] with a 5- and 10-year survival for the low- and high-risk groups of 92% and 85% and 65% and 42%, respectively.

SUPPORTING TREATMENT

Active and prolonged physical therapy is essential to accelerate neurologic recovery and avoid tendinous retractions in patients with severe motor impairment. Ankle foot orthotics combating equine gait are useful to facilitate walking and to diminish the risk of falling. Distal neuropathic pains should of course be treated. Devices facilitating breathing (continuous positive airway pressure) can be offered to patients with respiratory disorders. Psychological support is often necessary in this chronic disease with often a very slow improvement and an absence of a clear response to patients' questions by physicians who do not know well this complicated and very rare disease.

CONCLUDING REMARKS

In summary, important progress has been made in the management of POEMS syndrome since its first descriptions. Making the diagnosis remains a challenge because of its rarity, its polymorphic presentation, and the absence in many cases of a real tumoral disease. Measurement of VEGF and new imaging tools may help to make a rapid diagnosis essential to treat patients before severe neurologic impairment. A risk-adapted treatment should be given to patients, with often an excellent outcome. Further progress will come from a better understanding of its complex physiopathology.

REFERENCES

1. Li J, Zhang W, Jiao L, et al. Combination of melphalan and dexamethasone for patients with newly diagnosed POEMS syndrome. Blood 2011;117:6445–9.
2. Misawa S, Sato Y, Katayama K, et al. Safety and efficacy of thalidomide in patients with POEMS syndrome: a multicentre, randomised, double-blind, placebo-controlled trial. Lancet Neurol 2016;15:1129–37.
3. Jaccard A, Magy L. Thalidomide and POEMS syndrome: a cautious step forward. Lancet Neurol 2016;15:1104–5.
4. Merlini G, Stone MJ. Dangerous small B-cell clones. Blood 2006;108:2520–30.
5. Soubrier M, Labauge P, Jouanel P, et al. Restricted use of Vlambda genes in POEMS syndrome. Haematologica 2004;89:ECR02.
6. Abe D, Nakaseko C, Takeuchi M, et al. Restrictive usage of monoclonal immunoglobulin lambda light chain germline in POEMS syndrome. Blood 2008;112:836–9.
7. Aravamudan B, Tong C, Lacy MQ, et al. Immunoglobulin variable light chain restriction, cytokine expression and plasma cell-stromal cell interactions in POEMS syndrome patients. Blood 2008;112:2744.
8. Li J, Huang Z, Duan M-H, et al. Characterization of immunoglobulin λ light chain variable region (IGLV) gene and its relationship with clinical features in patients with POEMS syndrome. Ann Hematol 2012;91(8):1251–5.
9. Dao LN, Hanson CA, Dispenzieri A, et al. Bone marrow histopathology in POEMS syndrome: a distinctive combination of plasma cell, lymphoid and myeloid findings in 87 patients. Blood 2011;117:6438–44.
10. Wang C, Su W, Zhang W, et al. Serum immunoglobulin free light chain and heavy/light chain measurements in POEMS syndrome. Ann Hematol 2014;93:1201–6.
11. Pavord SR, Murphy PT, Mitchell VE. POEMS syndrome and Waldenstrom's macroglobulinaemia. J Clin Pathol 1996;49:181–2.
12. Dispenzieri A. POEMS syndrome. Blood Rev 2007;21:285–99.

13. Dispenzieri A. POEMS syndrome: 2017 update on diagnosis, risk stratification, and management. Am J Hematol 2017;92:814–29.
14. Suh YG, Suh CO, Kim JS, et al. Radiotherapy for solitary plasmacytoma of bone and soft tissue: outcomes and prognostic factors. Ann Hematol 2012;91: 1785–93.
15. Humeniuk MS, Gertz MA, Lacy MQ, et al. Outcomes of patients with POEMS syndrome treated initially with radiation. Blood 2013;122:66–73.
16. Kourelis TV, Buadi FK, Gertz MA, et al. Risk factors for and outcomes of patients with POEMS syndrome who experience progression after first-line treatment. Leukemia 2016;30:1079–85.
17. Suh YG, Kim YS, Suh CO, et al. The role of radiotherapy in the management of POEMS syndrome. Radiat Oncol 2014;9:265.
18. Jaccard A, Lazareth A, Karlin L, et al. A prospective phase II trial of lenalidomide and dexamethasone (LEN-DEX) in POEMS syndrome. Blood 2014;124:36.
19. Jaccard A, Royer B, Bordessoule D, et al. High-dose therapy and autologous blood stem cell transplantation in POEMS syndrome. Blood 2002;99:3057–9.
20. Dispenzieri A, Moreno-Aspitia A, Suarez GA, et al. Peripheral blood stem cell transplantation in 16 patients with POEMS syndrome, and a review of the literature. Blood 2004;104:3400–7.
21. D'Souza A, Lacy M, Gertz M, et al. Long-term outcomes after autologous stem cell transplantation for patients with POEMS syndrome (osteosclerotic myeloma): a single-center experience. Blood 2012;120:56–62.
22. Cook G, Iacobelli S, van Biezen A, et al. High-dose therapy and autologous stem cell transplantation in patients with POEMS syndrome: a retrospective study of the plasma cell disorder sub-committee of the Chronic Malignancy Working Party of the European Society for Blood & Marrow Transplantation. Haematologica 2017;102:160–7.
23. Dispenzieri A, Lacy MQ, Hayman SR, et al. Peripheral blood stem cell transplant for POEMS syndrome is associated with high rates of engraftment syndrome. Eur J Haematol 2008;80:397–406.
24. Nakaseko C, Ohwada C, Shimizu N, et al. Long-term outcomes of autologous stem cell transplantation for POEMS syndrome; a single center experience of 23 cases. Clin Lymphoma Myeloma Leuk 2013;13:S46–7.
25. Kim SY, Lee SA, Ryoo HM, et al. Thalidomide for POEMS syndrome. Ann Hematol 2006;85:545–6.
26. Dispenzieri A, Klein CJ, Mauermann ML. Lenalidomide therapy in a patient with POEMS syndrome. Blood 2007;110:1075–6.
27. Royer B, Merlusca L, Abraham J, et al. Efficacy of lenalidomide in POEMS syndrome: a retrospective study of 20 patients. Am J Hematol 2013;88:207–12.
28. Zagouri F, Kastritis E, Gavriatopoulou M, et al. Lenalidomide in patients with POEMS syndrome: a systematic review and pooled analysis. Leuk Lymphoma 2014;55:2018–23.
29. Sekiguchi Y, Misawa S, Shibuya K, et al. Ambiguous effects of anti-VEGF monoclonal antibody (bevacizumab) for POEMS syndrome. J Neurol Neurosurg Psychiatr 2013;84:1346–8.
30. Zeng K, Yang JR, Li J, et al. Effective induction therapy with subcutaneous administration of bortezomib for newly diagnosed POEMS syndrome: a case report and a review of the literature. Acta Haematol 2013;129:101–5.
31. Jouve P, Humbert M, Chauveheid MP. POEMS syndrome-related pulmonary hypertension is steroid-responsive. Respir Med 2007;101:353–5.

32. He H, Fu W, Du J, et al. Successful treatment of newly diagnosed POEMS syndrome with reduced-dose bortezomib based regimen. Br J Haematol 2017. [Epub ahead of print].

33. Dupont SA, Dispenzieri A, Mauermann ML, et al. Cerebral infarction in POEMS syndrome: incidence, risk factors, and imaging characteristics. Neurology 2009;73:1308–12.

34. Kawano Y, Nakama T, Hata H, et al. Successful treatment with rituximab and thalidomide of POEMS syndrome associated with Waldenstrom macroglobulinemia. J Neurol Sci 2010;15(297):101–4.

35. Terracciano C, Fiore S, Doldo E, et al. Inverse correlation between VEGF and soluble VEGF receptor 2 in POEMS with AIDP responsive to intravenous immunoglobulin. Muscle Nerve 2010;42:445–8.

36. D'Souza A, Hayman SR, Buadi F, et al. The utility of plasma vascular endothelial growth factor levels in the diagnosis and follow-up of patients with POEMS syndrome. Blood 2011;118:4663–5.

37. Dispenzieri A. Ushering in a new era for POEMS. Blood 2011;117:6405–6.

38. Graham RC, Hughes RAC. A modified peripheral neuropathy scale: the overall neuropathy limitations scale. J Neurol Neurosurg Psychiatry 2006;77:973–6.

39. Mudge S, Stott NS. Timed walking tests correlate with daily step activity in persons with stroke. Arch Phys Med Rehabil 2009;90:296–301.

40. Dispenzieri A, Kyle RA, Lacy MQ, et al. POEMS syndrome: definitions and long-term outcome. Blood 2003;101(7):2496–506.

41. Wang C, Huang XF, Cai QQ, et al. Prognostic study for overall survival in patients with newly diagnosed POEMS syndrome. Leukemia 2017;31:100–6.

42. Kourelis TV, Dispenzieri A. Validation of a prognostic score for patients with POEMS syndrome: a mayo clinic cohort. Leukemia 2017;31:1251.

The Peripheral Neuropathies of POEMS Syndrome and Castleman Disease

CrossMark

Michelle L. Mauermann, MD

KEYWORDS

- POEMS syndrome • POEMS neuropathy • Castleman disease
- Castleman neuropathy • Monoclonal gammopathy

KEY POINTS

- Polyneuropathy, organomegaly, endocrinopathy, monoclonal plasma cell-proliferative disorder, skin changes (POEMS) syndrome often presents with a peripheral neuropathy that is motor predominant with prominent lower limb weakness and atrophy.
- POEMS syndrome should be considered in patients with a diagnosis of chronic inflammatory demyelinating polyradiculoneuropathy that is resistant to standard therapy.
- Frequent neuropathic pain and absence of cranial nerve involvement in POEMS syndrome are helpful in distinguishing clinical characteristics from chronic inflammatory demyelinating polyradiculoneuropathy (CIDP).
- Peripheral neuropathy can occur in multicentric Castleman disease and is often a mild distal sensory neuropathy.

INTRODUCTION

Monoclonal gammopathies affect 3% to 4% of the population older than 50 years and affect more than 5% of the population older than 70 years.[1] They reflect a diverse group of disorders that share the secretion of monoclonal immunoglobulin produced by the bone marrow. These disorders include multiple myeloma; polyneuropathy, organomegaly, endocrinopathy, monoclonal protein, skin changes (POEMS) syndrome; Waldenström macroglobulinemia, light-chain amyloidosis; and monoclonal gammopathy of undetermined significance (MGUS). The most common neurologic complication is peripheral neuropathy. Monoclonal protein type and neuropathy pattern as well as the presence of other associated clinical features can aid in this determination. POEMS syndrome often presents with a subacute motor polyradiculoneuropathy, and the associated systemic features can be easily overlooked. The monoclonal protein is lambda in greater than 95% of cases, and its presence is a clue in patients who present with treatment-refractory chronic inflammatory

Department of Neurology, Mayo Clinic, 200 First Street Southwest, Rochester, MN 55905
E-mail address: Mauermann.Michelle@mayo.edu

Hematol Oncol Clin N Am 32 (2018) 153–163
https://doi.org/10.1016/j.hoc.2017.09.012
0889-8588/18/© 2017 Elsevier Inc. All rights reserved.

demyelinating polyradiculoneuropathy (CDIP). Castleman disease (CD) can be associated with POEMS syndrome but can also be present independent of POEMS syndrome. CD can be classified as unicentric or multicentric, with the latter associated with peripheral neuropathy. In contrast to POEMS syndrome, the neuropathy of CD is often a mild distal sensory neuropathy. The neuropathies associated with POEMS and CD are reviewed in detail.

POLYNEUROPATHY, ORGANOMEGALY, ENDOCRINOPATHY, MONOCLONAL PLASMA CELL-PROLIFERATIVE DISORDER, SKIN CHANGES (POEMS) SYNDROME
General

POEMS syndrome is a clonal plasma cell disorder that is described by the acronym in its name: polyneuropathy, organomegaly, endocrinopathy, monoclonal plasma cell-proliferative disorder, and skin changes. Other names used for POEMS syndrome include Takatsuki syndrome, Crow-Fukase syndrome, or osteosclerotic myeloma. There are many features associated with the syndrome, and the diagnostic criteria are listed in **Table 1**.[2] Monoclonal plasma cell-proliferative disorder and peripheral neuropathy are required for the diagnosis. One other major criterion, elevated vascular

Table 1 Criteria for the diagnosis of polyneuropathy, organomegaly, endocrinopathy, monoclonal protein, skin changes syndrome[a]	
Mandatory major criteria	1. Polyneuropathy (typically demyelinating) 2. Monoclonal plasma cell-proliferative disorder (almost always lambda)
Other major criteria (one required)	3. CD[a] 4. Sclerotic bone lesions 5. Vascular endothelial growth factor elevation
Minor criteria	6. Organomegaly (splenomegaly, hepatomegaly, or lymphadenopathy) 7. Extravascular volume overload (edema, pleural effusion, or ascites) 8. Endocrinopathy (adrenal, thyroid,[b] pituitary, gonadal, parathyroid, pancreatic[b]) 9. Skin changes (hyperpigmentation, hypertrichosis, glomeruloid hemangiomata, plethora, acrocyanosis, flushing, white nails) 10. Papilledema 11. Thrombocytosis/polycythemia[c]
Other symptoms and signs	Clubbing, weight loss, hyperhidrosis, pulmonary hypertension/restrictive lung disease, thrombotic diatheses, diarrhea, low vitamin B_{12} values

The diagnosis of POEMS syndrome is confirmed when both of the mandatory major criteria, one of the 3 other major criteria, and one of the 6 minor criteria are present.

[a] There is a CD variant of POEMS syndrome that occurs *without* evidence of a clonal plasma cell disorder that is not accounted for in this table. This entity should be considered separately.

[b] Because of the high prevalence of diabetes mellitus and thyroid abnormalities, this diagnosis alone is not sufficient to meet this minor criterion.

[c] Approximately 50% of patients will have bone marrow changes that distinguish it from a typical MGUS or myeloma bone marrow.[8] Anemia and/or thrombocytopenia are distinctively unusual in this syndrome unless CD is present.

From Dispenzieri A. POEMS syndrome: 2017 update on diagnosis, risk stratification, and management. Am J Hematol 2017;92(8):815; with permission.

endothelial growth factor (VEGF), CD, or sclerotic bone lesions, is also required. Patients are also required to have 2 minor criteria. These criteria include organomegaly (hepatomegaly, splenomegaly), lymphadenopathy, extravascular volume overload, endocrinopathy, skin changes, papilledema, or thrombocytosis/polycythemia.

Neuropathy Characteristics

Peripheral neuropathy is often the presenting or dominant clinical feature of POEMS syndrome and is required for the diagnosis. The neuropathy presents subacutely in a length-dependent manner with distal symmetric sensory symptoms (including tingling, burning) followed by weakness. It progresses proximally often into a polyradiculoneuropathy. Patients often have significant lower limb involvement with bilateral foot drop and lower limb atrophy and can be so severe that patients require a wheelchair or even become bedbound.[3,4] Patients are often areflexic. The neuropathy is often mistaken for CIDP because of the presentation of a subacute motor-predominant polyradiculoneuropathy. This presentation often leads to a delay in diagnosis and development of worsened disability and development of other multiorgan involvement.[5] **Table 2** details features distinguishing POEMS syndrome and CIDP. Neuropathic pain in the lower limbs can be a helpful distinguishing feature, as it is present in 76% of patients with POEMS syndrome and only 7% of patients with CIDP ($P<.001$).[5] Patients with POEMS syndrome also rarely have cranial nerve involvement (2%); therefore, its presence would suggest an alternative diagnosis.[5]

Evaluation

In the evaluation of patients with a CIDP-like illness, especially when refractory to typical treatment (intravenous immunoglobulin, plasma exchange, corticosteroids), it is important to test for a monoclonal protein. In POEMS syndrome, the plasma cells

Table 2
Neuropathy and electrodiagnostic characteristics differentiating polyneuropathy, organomegaly, endocrinopathy, monoclonal plasma cell-proliferative disorder, skin changes syndrome and chronic inflammatory demyelinating polyradiculoneuropathy

	POEMS Syndrome	CIDP
Neuropathy Characteristics		
Subacute onset	+++	+++
Motor predominant	+++	+++
Lower extremity atrophy	+++	+
Pain	+++	+/−
Cranial nerve palsy	+/−	+
EDX Characteristics		
Sural sparing	+/−	++
Conduction block	+/−	+
Temporal dispersion	+	+
Laboratory Characteristics		
Monoclonal protein (lambda)	+++	+/−
Elevated VEGF	+++	+/−
Thrombocytosis	++	+/−

Abbreviations: EDX, electrodiagnostic study; +++, greater than 50% of cases; ++, 25% to 50% of cases; +, 10% to 25% of cases; +/−, less than 10% of cases.

are lambda light-chain restricted in greater than 95% of cases.[6] Lambda-free light chains are usually elevated (90%); however, an abnormal free light-chain ratio is seen in a minority of patients (18%).[7] A serum monoclonal protein is absent in 24% to 54% of patients, and these patients may have a solitary plasmacytoma.[6] Iliac crest biopsy demonstrates lymphoid aggregates (49%) with plasma cells rimming (97%) that are usually lambda positive with megakaryocyte hyperplasia (54%) and megakaryocyte clustering (93%).[8] There is no evidence of clonal plasma cells in one-third of patients, and these patients usually present with solitary or multiple solitary plasmacytomas.[8] The median percent of plasma cells is less than 5%, usually in a background of increased polytypic plasma cells. Thrombocytosis is seen in 54% of patients with POEMS syndrome and can help differentiate from CIDP, as it is rare in that condition (1.5%).[9] VEGF is the cytokine that correlates best with disease activity but does not correlate with the severity of the neuropathy.[4] VEGF increases vascular permeability, targets endothelial cells, and is important in angiogenesis; however, it may not be the driving force of the disease. A plasma VEGF level of 200 pg/mL or greater has a specificity of 95% and sensitivity of 68%.[10] A serum VEGF of 1920 pg/mL or greater has a specificity of 98% and sensitivity of 73%.[11] interleukin (IL) 12 levels are also often elevated.[12] Cerebrospinal fluid evaluation demonstrates a normal cell count with elevated protein (albuminocytologic dissociation).

Electrodiagnostic Characteristics

Nerve conduction studies and electromyography are necessary to characterize the peripheral neuropathy. In POEMS syndrome, the initial findings on nerve conduction studies support a primary demyelinating process with secondary axonal injury.[13] There is slowing of motor and sensory nerve conduction velocities and prolongation of motor and sensory distal latencies and prolonged F-wave latencies implying uniform slowing along the nerve.[3] Conduction block is seen in 6.7% and temporal dispersion in 13.3% of patients. Lower greater than upper limb compound muscle action potential amplitudes and sensory nerve action potential (SNAP) amplitudes are reduced implying axonal loss. The presence of sural sparing (present sural SNAP with absent median and ulnar SNAPs) was not seen in a published series of patients with POEMS syndrome.[3] Needle electromyography demonstrates length-dependent neurogenic abnormalities but with proximal involvement consistent with a polyradiculoneuropathy. The blink reflex is a monosynaptic reflex of cranial nerves V and VII. The R1 latency has been shown to be a sensitive and specific marker of demyelination in inherited neuropathies.[14] The R1 latency of the blink reflex is prolonged in 65% of patients with POEMS syndrome, consistent with a demyelinating process.[15] It is especially helpful in severe POEMS syndrome cases whereby the limb nerve conduction studies are severely reduced or absent. Compared with patients with CIDP, nerve conduction studies in POEMS syndrome demonstrate greater axonal loss (reduction of motor amplitudes especially in the lower limbs and increased fibrillation potentials) and more uniform slowing (greater slowing of the intermediate nerve segments, less prolonged distal latencies, and higher terminal latency indices in POEMS syndrome). Terminal latency index is another measure used to evaluate slowing involving the distal nerve segment.

Radiologic Features

Metastatic bone survey should be performed to look for osteosclerotic lesions, which occur in approximately 95% of patients. These lesions can be confused with benign bone islands, aneurysmal bone cysts, nonossifying fibromas, and fibrous dysplasia.[16] Computed skeletal survey is more sensitive in identifying sclerotic lesions and in one series of 24 patients, all patients had sclerotic bone lesions, the majority being less than 1 cm, which were not identified radiographically.[17] Fluorodeoxyglucose uptake occurs in lesions 2 cm or greater with a lytic component.[18] Nerve imaging may show abnormalities that are not unique to POEMS syndrome and are reported in other immune polyradiculoneuropathies. One series of 6 patients who had MRI of the lumbosacral spine showed definite enhancement of multiple lumbosacral nerve roots and possible root enlargement.[19]

Pathologic Features

The pathophysiology of the neuropathy in POEMS syndrome is incompletely understood. One early finding is the alteration in sodium and potassium channels present in the nodes of Ranvier and axon.[20] Increased VEGF levels have been associated with vasculopathy of the vasa nervorum.[21,22] The imbalance of increased VEGF and decreased serum erythropoietin is thought to increase neovascularization and induce functional alterations in the vessel wall that lead to increased permeability and edema.[23] A large series of nerve biopsy findings of patients with POEMS syndrome were compared with CIDP.[24] Patients with POEMS syndrome demonstrated increased demyelination and axonal degeneration, the latter of which was greater than in patients with CIDP (**Fig. 1**). The numbers of small epineurial blood vessels were increased, and a cutoff of greater than 120 epineurial vessels best differentiated these conditions (specificity of 77%, sensitivity of 54%) (**Fig. 2**). Patients with POEMS syndrome have less endoneurial mononuclear inflammation, and large onion bulbs were not seen.

Treatment

Treatment of the neuropathy in POEMS syndrome involves treating the underlying plasma cell disorder. The neuropathy has not been studied systematically in response

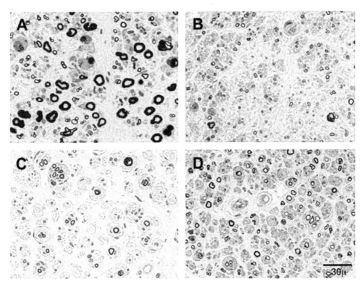

Fig. 1. Semithin epoxy transverse section from POEMS syndrome (*A, B*) and CIDP (*C, D*) biopsies (original magnification ×634). The biopsies show decreased density of myelinated fibers, active axonal degeneration, and lack of onion bulbs in the POEMS syndrome (*A, B*) and multiple large onion bulbs, decreased number of large myelinated fibers, and regenerating clusters present in the CIDP biopsies (*C, D*) (methylene blue). (*From* Piccione EA, Engelstad J, Dyck PJ, et al. Nerve pathologic features differentiate POEMS syndrome from CIDP. Acta Neuropathol Commun 2016;4(1):116; with permission.)

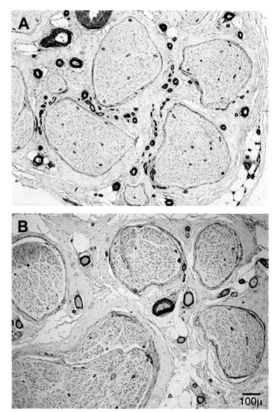

Fig. 2. Smooth muscle actin (SMACTIN, original magnification ×80) paraffin cross section from POEMS syndrome (*A*) and CIDP (*B*) biopsies (80×). There are increased numbers of small epineurial blood vessels in POEMS syndrome (*A*) compared with CIDP (*B*). (*From* Piccione EA, Engelstad J, Dyck PJ, et al. Nerve pathologic features differentiate POEMS syndrome from CIDP. Acta Neuropathol Commun 2016;4(1):116; with permission.)

to many of the treatments for POEMS syndrome. There is no agreed upon method to assess the response to treatment. Most studies have used a 1-point improvement in the Overall Neuropathy Limitation Scale. Using this approach, improvements have been seen with melphalan,[25] lenalidomide,[26] and bortezomib.[27] It is not clear how these treatments compare with one another or whether they are superior to autologous stem cell transplant. There have been 2 studies evaluating the effect of autologous stem cell transplant (ASCT) on the peripheral neuropathy. An initial study of 9 patients demonstrated improvement in the neuropathy within months and substantial improvements by 6 months.[28] Three wheelchair-bound patients regained the ability to walk at 6 months. The neuropathy continued to show improvement as far as 4 years following ASCT, and no patient showed worsening. A larger study retrospectively evaluated 60 patients who underwent ASCT at a single institution.[4] There was an improvement in the Neuropathy Impairment Score and modified Rankin Score at 1 year and at the final follow-up (median 61 months) (**Figs. 3** and **4**). The improvement correlated with the decline in VEGF levels. There was an improvement in upper limb motor amplitudes. Nearly half of the patients needed a wheelchair before treatment, and all but one was able to walk within 1 year following ASCT. Further studies with direct comparison of immunomodulatory drugs (IMiDs) and proteasome inhibitors with ASCT are

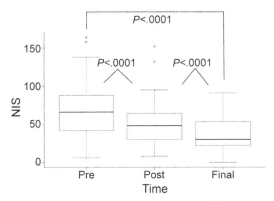

Fig. 3. Improvement in neuropathy impairment score (NIS) following autologous stem cell transplantation. Pre, prior to transplantation; Post, first followup, median 12 months; Final, last followup, median 49 months. (*From* Karam C, Klein CJ, Dispenzieri A, et al. Polyneuropathy improvement following autologous stem cell transplantation for POEMS syndrome. Neurology 2015;84(19):1984; with permission.)

needed to determine the most appropriate therapy in newly diagnosed and relapsed patients.

CASTLEMAN DISEASE
General

CD is a rare lymphoproliferative disorder characterized by enlarged lymph nodes and a wide spectrum of clinical manifestations. The clinical phenotype is driven by whether the lymphadenopathy is unicentric (confined to one region) or multicentric. Those with multicentric disease will most often present with constitutional symptoms and have palpable disease along with a variety of systemic symptoms, including peripheral neuropathy.[29] Peripheral neuropathy occurs in approximately 27% of patients with CD.[30,31] The presence of peripheral neuropathy is important in the classification of the disease because those with neuropathy tend to have relatively different

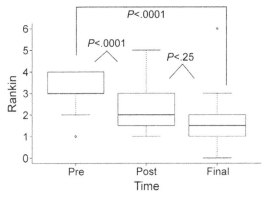

Fig. 4. Improvement in modified Rankin Scale (mRS) score following autologous stem cell transplantation. Pre, prior to transplantation; Post, first followup, median 12 months; Final, last followup, median 61 months. (*From* Karam C, Klein CJ, Dispenzieri A, et al. Polyneuropathy improvement following autologous stem cell transplantation for POEMS syndrome. Neurology 2015;84(19):1984; with permission.)

characteristics and might require a different treatment approach.[31–33] The peripheral neuropathy in CD has been reported with all histopathologic types, including plasma cell, hyaline vascular, and mixed.

Neuropathy Characteristics

The neuropathy associated with CD presents most commonly in the sixth decade. In patients without coexisting POEMS syndrome, the neuropathy typically presents with distal lower limb numbness. Approximately half of patients report positive sensory symptoms, such as tingling or burning, or motor symptoms, such as weakness[30] Pain is often absent. The neurologic examination demonstrates length-dependent sensory deficits in the lower limbs rarely with objective weakness. When CD is present in the setting of POEMS syndrome, the neuropathy is similar to that of POEMS syndrome with a motor and sensory polyneuropathy or polyradiculoneuropathy but less severe. More than half of patients report burning, shooting, or stabbing pain, often requiring neuropathic pain medications (**Table 3**).[30]

Evaluation

There is no plasma cell disorder by definition in those cases of CD without coexisting POEMS syndrome. In those that occur in the setting of POEMS syndrome, the plasma cell disorder is almost always lambda restricted and of non–immunoglobulin M isotype. VEGF levels are often elevated irrespective of the presence of POEMS syndrome, and the degree of abnormality does not predict the specific condition.[30] IL-6 levels may also be elevated and are related to the pathogenesis of the disease. Thrombocytosis may be seen in those without POEMS syndrome but is more common if POEMS syndrome is present.[9] CD can also be associated with human immunodeficiency virus (HIV). In all patients who are HIV positive and nearly half of HIV-negative patients, the lymph nodes are positive for human herpesvirus-8 (HHV-8).[34–39]

Electrophysiologic Features

The nerve conduction studies and electromyography in CD also support a primary demyelinating process. In addition, there is evidence of secondary axonal loss, but

Table 3
Neuropathy symptoms at presentation of Castleman disease versus polyneuropathy, organomegaly, endocrinopathy, monoclonal plasma cell-proliferative disorder, skin changes syndrome

Parameter	CD-PN (n = 7)	CD-POEMS (n = 20)	POEMS (n = 122)	P Values
Duration of neuropathic symptoms (mo)	15 (12–72)	48 (5–132)	15 (1–120)	.0058
Weakness, n (%)	3 (43)	14 (70)	113 (93)	.0004
Numbness, n (%)	6 (86)	19 (95)	97 (80)	NS
Paresthesias, n (%)	4 (57)	17 (85)	89 (73)	NS
Neuropathic pain, n (%)	0 (0)	11 (55)	67 (55)	.0327
Neuropathic pain medication, n (%)	1 (14.3)	10 (50)	55 (45)	NS
Opioid use, n (%)	0 (0)	3 (15)	30 (25)	NS

Abbreviations: NS, greater than .05; PN, peripheral neuropathy.
From Naddaf E, Dispenzieri A, Mandrekar J, et al. Clinical spectrum of Castleman disease-associated neuropathy. Neurology 2016;87(23):2459; with permission.

there is a spectrum of severity. In those without POEMS syndrome, the nerve conduction studies are mainly restricted to reduced sensory amplitudes.[30] These patients have the mildest degree of axonal loss, followed by CD with POEMS syndrome and lastly POEMS syndrome without CD.

Pathologic Features

Likely because of the mild nature of the neuropathy associated with CD without POEMS syndrome, there are no reports of nerve biopsies in these patients. In those with coexisting POEMS syndrome, the nerve biopsy shows findings are as described earlier in this review.

Treatment

The treatment of CD can include anti–IL-6 (siltuximab), chemotherapy, corticosteroids, antiviral drugs to block HHV-8 or HIV activity if present, or thalidomide. Further study is needed to determine the neuropathy response to treatment in these patients.

SUMMARY

Peripheral neuropathy is required for the diagnosis of POEMS syndrome and is often the presenting and dominant feature of the illness. It is typically a subacute, painful motor-predominant demyelinating polyradiculoneuropathy and causes significant morbidity. In contrast, peripheral neuropathy in CD is only present in approximately one-quarter of patients and is often mild in severity. It is typically a painless distal sensory demyelinating neuropathy. Elevated VEGF can be seen in both conditions, and the levels do not predict the underlying disease. Although there are several treatments in POEMS syndrome that have been shown to be effective for the treatment of the neuropathy associated with POEMS syndrome, there is no current evidence demonstrating an improvement in neuropathy with known treatments of CD.

REFERENCES

1. Kyle RA, Therneau TM, Rajkumar SV, et al. Prevalence of monoclonal gammopathy of undetermined significance. N Engl J Med 2006;354(13):1362–9.
2. Dispenzieri A. POEMS syndrome: 2017 update on diagnosis, risk stratification, and management. Am J Hematol 2017;92(8):814–29.
3. Mauermann ML, Sorenson EJ, Dispenzieri A, et al. Uniform demyelination and more severe axonal loss distinguish POEMS syndrome from CIDP. J Neurol Neurosurg Psychiatry 2012;83(5):480–6.
4. Karam C, Klein CJ, Dispenzieri A, et al. Polyneuropathy improvement following autologous stem cell transplantation for POEMS syndrome. Neurology 2015; 84(19):1981–7.
5. Nasu S, Misawa S, Sekiguchi Y, et al. Different neurological and physiological profiles in POEMS syndrome and chronic inflammatory demyelinating polyneuropathy. J Neurol Neurosurg Psychiatry 2012;83(5):476–9.
6. Dispenzieri A. POEMS syndrome: update on diagnosis, risk-stratification, and management. Am J Hematol 2015;90(10):951–62.
7. Stankowski-Drengler T, Gertz MA, Katzmann JA, et al. Serum immunoglobulin free light chain measurements and heavy chain isotype usage provide insight into disease biology in patients with POEMS syndrome. Am J Hematol 2010; 85(6):431–4.

8. Dao LN, Hanson CA, Dispenzieri A, et al. Bone marrow histopathology in POEMS syndrome: a distinctive combination of plasma cell, lymphoid, and myeloid findings in 87 patients. Blood 2011;117(24):6438–44.

9. Naddaf E, Dispenzieri A, Mandrekar J, et al. Thrombocytosis distinguishes POEMS syndrome from chronic inflammatory demyelinating polyneuropathy. Muscle Nerve 2015;52(4):658–9.

10. D'Souza A, Hayman SR, Buadi F, et al. The utility of plasma vascular endothelial growth factor levels in the diagnosis and follow-up of patients with POEMS syndrome. Blood 2011;118(17):4663–5.

11. Wang C, Zhou YL, Cai H, et al. Markedly elevated serum total N-terminal propeptide of type I collagen is a novel marker for the diagnosis and follow up of patients with POEMS syndrome. Haematologica 2014;99(6):e78–80.

12. Kanai K, Sawai S, Sogawa K, et al. Markedly upregulated serum interleukin-12 as a novel biomarker in POEMS syndrome. Neurology 2012;79(6):575–82.

13. Liu M, Zou Z, Guan Y, et al. Motor nerve conduction study and muscle strength in newly diagnosed POEMS syndrome. Muscle Nerve 2015;51(1):19–23.

14. Wang W, Litchy WJ, Mandrekar J, et al. Blink reflex role in algorithmic genetic testing of inherited polyneuropathies. Muscle Nerve 2017;55(3):316–22.

15. Wang W, Litchy WJ, Mauermann ML, et al. Blink R1 latency utility in diagnosis and treatment assessment of polyradiculoneuropathy-organomegaly-endocrinopathy-monoclonal protein-skin changes and chronic inflammatory demyelinating polyradiculoneuropathy. Muscle Nerve 2017. [Epub ahead of print].

16. Clark MS, Howe BM, Glazebrook KN, et al. Osteolytic-variant POEMS syndrome: an uncommon presentation of "osteosclerotic" myeloma. Skeletal Radiol 2017; 46(6):817–23.

17. Glazebrook K, Guerra Bonilla FL, Johnson A, et al. Computed tomography assessment of bone lesions in patients with POEMS syndrome. Eur Radiol 2015;25(2):497–504.

18. Pan Q, Li J, Li F, et al. Characterizing POEMS syndrome with 18F-FDG PET/CT. J Nucl Med 2015;56(9):1334–7.

19. Li Y, Valent J, Soltanzadeh P, et al. Diagnostic challenges in POEMS syndrome presenting with polyneuropathy: a case series. J Neurol Sci 2017;378:170–4.

20. Hashimoto R, Koike H, Takahashi M, et al. Uncompacted myelin lamellae and nodal ion channel disruption in POEMS syndrome. J Neuropathol Exp Neurol 2015;74(12):1127–36.

21. Watanabe O, Maruyama I, Arimura K, et al. Overproduction of vascular endothelial growth factor/vascular permeability factor is causative in Crow-Fukase (POEMS) syndrome. Muscle Nerve 1998;21(11):1390–7.

22. Watanabe O, Arimura K, Kitajima I, et al. Greatly raised vascular endothelial growth factor (VEGF) in POEMS syndrome. Lancet 1996;347(9002):702.

23. Scarlato M, Previtali SC, Carpo M, et al. Polyneuropathy in POEMS syndrome: role of angiogenic factors in the pathogenesis. Brain 2005;128(Pt 8):1911–20.

24. Piccione EA, Engelstad J, Dyck PJ, et al. Nerve pathologic features differentiate POEMS syndrome from CIDP. Acta Neuropathol Commun 2016;4(1):116.

25. Li J, Zhang W, Jiao L, et al. Combination of melphalan and dexamethasone for patients with newly diagnosed POEMS syndrome. Blood 2011;117(24):6445–9.

26. Zagouri F, Kastritis E, Gavriatopoulou M, et al. Lenalidomide in patients with POEMS syndrome: a systematic review and pooled analysis. Leuk Lymphoma 2014;55(9):2018–23.

27. He H, Fu W, Du J, et al. Successful treatment of newly diagnosed POEMS syn-drome with reduced-dose bortezomib based regimen. Br J Haematol 2017. [Epub ahead of print].
28. Kuwabara S. New strategy of treatment for POEMS syndrome–autologous periph-eral blood stem cell transplantation and thalidomide therapy. Brain Nerve 2008; 60(6):627–33 [in Japanese].
29. Dispenzieri A, Armitage JO, Loe MJ, et al. The clinical spectrum of Castleman's disease. Am J Hematol 2012;87(11):997–1002.
30. Naddaf E, Dispenzieri A, Mandrekar J, et al. Clinical spectrum of Castleman disease-associated neuropathy. Neurology 2016;87(23):2457–62.
31. Nakanishi T, Sobue I, Toyokura Y, et al. The Crow-Fukase syndrome: a study of 102 cases in Japan. Neurology 1984;34(6):712–20.
32. Hineman VL, Phyliky RL, Banks PM. Angiofollicular lymph node hyperplasia and peripheral neuropathy: association with monoclonal gammopathy. Mayo Clin Proc 1982;57(6):379–82.
33. Menke DM, Camoriano JK, Banks PM. Angiofollicular lymph node hyperplasia: a comparison of unicentric, multicentric, hyaline vascular, and plasma cell types of disease by morphometric and clinical analysis. Mod Pathol 1992;5(5):525–30.
34. Soulier J, Grollet L, Oksenhendler E, et al. Kaposi's sarcoma-associated herpes-virus-like DNA sequences in multicentric Castleman's disease. Blood 1995;86(4): 1276–80.
35. Chadburn A, Cesarman E, Nador RG, et al. Kaposi's sarcoma-associated herpesvirus sequences in benign lymphoid proliferations not associated with hu-man immunodeficiency virus. Cancer 1997;80(4):788–97.
36. Parravicini C, Corbellino M, Paulli M, et al. Expression of a virus-derived cytokine, KSHV vIL-6, in HIV-seronegative Castleman's disease. Am J Pathol 1997;151(6): 1517–22.
37. O'Leary J, Kennedy M, Howells D, et al. Cellular localisation of HHV-8 in Castle-man's disease: is there a link with lymph node vascularity? Mol Pathol 2000;53(2): 69–76.
38. Suda T, Katano H, Delsol G, et al. HHV-8 infection status of AIDS-unrelated and AIDS-associated multicentric Castleman's disease. Pathol Int 2001;51(9):671–9.
39. Amin HM, Medeiros LJ, Manning JT, et al. Dissolution of the lymphoid follicle is a feature of the HHV8+ variant of plasma cell Castleman's disease. Am J Surg Pathol 2003;27(1):91–100.

Moving?

Make sure your subscription moves with you!

To notify us of your new address, find your **Clinics Account Number** (located on your mailing label above your name), and contact customer service at:

Email: journalscustomerservice-usa@elsevier.com

800-654-2452 (subscribers in the U.S. & Canada)
314-447-8871 (subscribers outside of the U.S. & Canada)

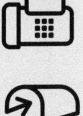

Fax number: 314-447-8029

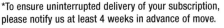

Elsevier Health Sciences Division
Subscription Customer Service
3251 Riverport Lane
Maryland Heights, MO 63043

*To ensure uninterrupted delivery of your subscription, please notify us at least 4 weeks in advance of move.

Printed and bound by CPI Group (UK) Ltd, Croydon, CR0 4YY

03/10/2024

01040391-0017